Collaborative Therapeutic Neuropsychological Assessment

Tad T. Gorske · Steven R. Smith

Collaborative Therapeutic Neuropsychological Assessment

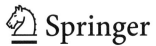 Springer

Tad T. Gorske
Department of Physical Medicine
  and Rehabilitation
University of Pittsburgh
  School of Medicine
Pittsburgh, PA
gorskett@upmc.edu

Steven R. Smith
Department of Counseling, Clinical
  and School Psychology
University of California
Santa Barbara, CA
ssmith@education.ucsb.edu

ISBN: 978-0-387-75425-3   e-ISBN: 978-0-387-75426-0
DOI 10.1007/978-0-387-75426-0

Library of Congress Control Number: 2008936883

Printed on acid-free paper

springer.com

Foreword

It is my great pleasure to introduce this important and timely book. Collaborative and therapeutic assessment methods are becoming better known in the area of personality assessment, but they are still unfamiliar to many practicing neuropsychologists, in spite of the work of Luria and Vygotsky, yet this need no longer be the case.

In this clear and extremely useful volume, Tad Gorske and Steve Smith teach neuropsychological assessors to engage their clients as full collaborators in the assessment process and to discuss assessment findings in ways that clients will find useful and transformative. This book has the potential to spur a paradigm shift in neuropsychological assessment, much as the work of Constance Fischer and others are doing in clinical personality assessment.

This is not to imply that Smith and Gorske have simply imported their principles and methods from collaborative personality assessment. They have integrated the work of Carl Rogers in much of their thinking, and their use of the principles and techniques of Motivational Interviewing is unique and leads to many useful innovations. The authors also draw on their own research and clinical experience in offering detailed guidelines on how to make neuropsychological assessment a self-enhancing experience for clients; this gives a sense of authenticity to their suggestions.

I particularly liked the careful attention paid to different ways of conducting the initial clinical interview and the sample dialogue detailing conversations between assessors and clients, which were engaging and educational. The detailed instructions on how to give feedback were marvelous, and the clinical examples brought this section to life. Also, I have never seen a more respectful set of guidelines offered for handling recommendations with clients at the end of an assessment. Any clinician reading this book will come away with specific language and techniques for discussing sensitive information with clients, even if that clinician never administers a single neuropsychological test.

In summary, I am grateful for having read this book, and I highly recommend it to novice and experienced psychological assessors alike. I look forward eagerly to seeing the impact of Gorske and Smith's work on the field of neuropsychological assessment.

Center for Therapeutic Assessment, Austin, TX   Stephen E. Finn

Preface

I had a wonderful experience during the Society for Personality Assessment Annual Convention in Spring 2006. About 6 months prior, while starting up the study, Effects of Cognitive Test Feedback on Patient Adherence, on a whim I decided to email Dr. Stephen Finn and ask him what he had been doing with Therapeutic Assessment recently and if he knew of any applications to neuropsychology. Up to that point, I had completed a feasibility study examining cognitive test feedback outcomes and was in the process of beginning a more formal pilot study. My experiences of sending such emails to other professionals were mixed at best, usually responded to with little interest or no response at all. However, Stephen Finn's response to me was enthusiastic and welcoming, and it was then that he helped me get in touch with Dr. Steven Smith at U.C. Santa Barbara and Dr. Diane Engelman at the Center for Collaborative Psychology and Psychiatry in Sonoma, California. From there we began a series of email communications that led to our first presentation at the Society for Personality Assessment in 2006, with Stephen Finn as our discussant. It was during that convention that Stephen said something to me that has been a consistent motivator in my life. He said, and I'm paraphrasing, that we (Steve Smith, Diane, and I) are where he and Connie (referring to Dr. Constance Fischer from Duquesne University) were about 20 years ago. Given the huge impact Therapeutic and Collaborative Psychological Assessment has had on the field, I considered that a major compliment. From that point, we have continually worked to develop and crystallize collaborative neuropsychological assessment methods.

Another story relates to how we came up with the name, Collaborative Therapeutic Neuropsychological Assessment. During our preparations for the first presentation in San Diego, Steve Smith and I had been going back and forth about what we should call ourselves. Steve was inclined toward Collaborative Neuropsychological Assessment while I was inclined toward Therapeutic Neuropsychological Assessment. It was Diane who chimed in and in her gentle and wise way, emailed both of us and said, "Thank you both for your efforts with thoughtful wording and sensitivity to the various aspects of *collaborative therapeutic neuropsychological assessment* and our working together as a team." (Personal Communication, September 22, 2005). The name stuck.

From that point on, CTNA has garnished support from members of the Society for Personality Assessment, the Pennsylvania Psychological Association, and neuropsychologists who have requested information about the work via personal communications and listserve correspondence. However, all of us realize that we are doing something different, innovative, and outside the mainstream of neuropsychology. This despite the fact that authors have been saying for 20 years or more that a neuropsychological assessment and feedback method is important and necessary. However, to date, no solid conceptual framework or model has been developed. We hope to fill this gap with CTNA and encourage others to read our work, use, and adapt it to their own needs and investigate its effects on patient satisfaction and outcomes.

We welcome all those who are interested in collaborative and patient-centered assessment and feedback methods to read and use this book in their own practice or research. We would caution that this book will not discuss basic methods of neuropsychological assessment interviewing, testing, and interpretation. It is assumed that readers will be well versed in these methods, and there are many other authoritative books describing these techniques and theories. Thus, the language in this book is used under the assumption that the reader understands neuropsychological assessment terminology and is familiar with various types of neuropsychological assessment cases. Readers who are less experienced in these areas may find some cases and terminology confusing and are referred to review references in neuropsychological assessment methods and cases provided at the end of the book.

One final note regarding the case studies interspersed throughout the book. Each of these cases represent actual patient experiences with important identifying information and details omitted or significantly modified to protect confidentiality. In some cases, the clinical information represents an amalgamation of similar patient cases; therefore, similarities to an actual person known to the reader is most likely coincidence or simply a reflection of common human experiences.

Pittsburgh, PA, USA   Tad T. Gorske, Ph.D.

Acknowledgments

We are indebted to the support and open arms of members of the Society for Personality Assessment, including Drs. Stephen Finn, Connie Fischer, and Leonard Handler, who have chaired our symposiums for the last 3 years and have offered numerous words of encouragement and support. We are most indebted to Dr. Diane Engelman. She has been a member of our CTNA team and is a gentle yet strong voice in her contributions to CTNA methods.

We want to thank members of the Pennsylvania Psychological Association who have provided a forum for disseminating CTNA and the members who have embraced it with open arms. In particular I would like to thank Dr. Mick Sittig, a rehabilitation psychologist at ReMed in Pittsburgh, Pennsylvania. Mick has been an ardent supporter of CTNA, and his excitement and enthusiasm has continued to motivate me to expand and develop this work.

We would like to also thank Dr. Christopher Ryan at the University of Pittsburgh School of Medicine. Dr. Ryan is the man who encouraged and supported my (Dr. Gorske's) efforts to develop CTNA methods. It was Dr. Ryan's belief in my abilities and potential that allowed me to think "outside the box" and continually develop the methods to their current form. We would also like to thank Dr. Dennis Daley at the University of Pittsburgh, Addiction Medicine Services, for providing resources and support for developing CTNA.

This work is partially supported by a grant from the National Institute on Drug Abuse DA017273-01A1.

Contents

Chapter 1
Challenges for Clinical Neuropsychology

The following examples are composites of possible neuropsychological assessment cases. These cases are composites in order to protect the identity of patients and the treating providers.

Case Examples

Case #1: A 54-year-old female patient is referred for neuropsychological testing by her neurologist after suffering a stroke. Prior to the stroke the patient was a high-functioning professional, active in her community, and raising three children. The patient's primary complaints were an inability to concentrate, focus, and clouding in her cognition. She also has problems with her speech in that she cannot express herself as easily and often seems detached and less emotionally expressive than she used to be. Additionally, her husband has pointed out that she seems to forget the names of things. Although she understands that she has had a stroke, she doesn't know what this means for her ability to function at work, which she takes a great deal of pride in. Her neurologist refers her for a neuropsychological assessment. When she asks what that means, she is told that it's a series of tests to see how she is functioning. She is even more confused because she has already received a series of tests including blood work and an electroencephalogram, and she has a prescription for an MRI. So what more is this test going to tell her, and why does she have to go? She contacts the psychologist whom the neurologist referred her to. Upon meeting the psychologist, she is immediately asked a series of questions about her personal life, daily habits, routines, ability to function at work and home, and others. She asks why this information is important, and the psychologist tells her that it's all part of a comprehensive evaluation. She is given a couple of self-report measures that ask her questions about how she is feeling and her sleep habits, eating habits, energy level, toileting and bathing habits, and others. She answers them but is unsure what the tests are supposed to measure. Afterward, she is asked more questions such as "what is the date, day, month, year, city we are in, county?" and others.

T.T. Gorske, S.R. Smith, *Collaborative Therapeutic Neuropsychological Assessment*,
DOI: 10.1007/978-0-387-75426-0_1, © Springer Science+Business Media, LLC 2009

Again confused, the patient asks why these questions are important. The psychologist smiles, writes some notes, and instructs her to give her best effort.

Afterward, she is given a series of tasks to do, remember stories, make lists of words, draw a picture, put blocks together, and many others. The testing is long and tiring. She begins to get a headache. It seems like it takes forever, but the psychologist keeps telling her to relax and give her best effort. Finally, after five exhausting hours, the testing is complete. The psychologist tells her that a report will be ready in about two or three weeks and will be sent to her neurologist. The patient never sees or hears from the psychologist again. She contacts her neurologist to find out about the results. She is told that the neurologist is busy with patients and that she will be scheduled in one month.

Case #2: An elderly woman, who has been experiencing symptoms of depression, decreased concentration and memory, anhedonia, and multiple medical complaints, is referred by her primary care physician to a psychologist for an evaluation. Her grown daughter accompanies her to attend the evaluation with the psychologist, who conducts interviews and tests. The daughter and her mother do not hear anything until four weeks later when they meet with the mother's physician, who received the test results. The physician states that the elderly mother has Alzheimer's disease and needs to be placed on Aricept. The daughter, in shock, demands to see the report. The physician gives her the report that consists of a psychosocial history, paragraphs of psychological jargon, a bunch of numbers, and then conclusions and recommendations that state "Probable Alzheimer's dementia." "Initiate treatment with a cholinesterase inhibitor." The daughter asks the physician what all the jargon and numbers mean, but he is unable to answer her.

Case #3: A man in his early 30s has changed his career aspirations and decided to become a pilot. After going through the appropriate training, he begins the process of taking all the required medical evaluations and tests. In his teen years, the man was arrested for an event involving alcohol and was ordered to attend drug and alcohol classes. Although there were no prior problems, the regulations from the FAA required that he undergo a comprehensive drug and alcohol evaluation including personality and neuropsychological testing. The man denied any abusive use of alcohol or any other substances, and for all intensive purposes, led a reasonably clean life, married, and had children. Nervous about the evaluation, he meets with the psychologist for an entire day, undergoing a psychosocial history evaluation and cognitive and personality tests. He was nervous partly due to his history of being arrested for underage drinking but also because there was a brief period in his life when he was depressed and received psychotherapy. After undergoing about eight hours of interviews and tests, the man leaves exhausted and anxious about what the results might mean. One month later he is called for a meeting with the primary medical evaluator. He is told that his approval for a pilot's license is delayed because the results of his tests indicated an "area of concern." He is given no further information.

Case #4: A woman in her late 30s is referred for a neuropsychological evaluation to assess whether the cognitive problems she is experiencing may have an organic basis or they are related to a diagnosed psychiatric disorder. The psychologist she is referred to conducts a thorough initial evaluation, including a review of all available medical and previous mental health treatment records. He conducts a comprehensive evaluation that includes neuropsychological tests, personality tests, and other self-report measures. Upon completing the evaluation, the psychologist generates a comprehensive report that is mailed to the referral source, with proper consents, and to the patient. About three weeks later, he receives a phone call from the patient stating that she is contacting her attorney and the ethics board because she disagreed with the report and because impressions were never shared, and consequently she had no say in the findings prior to the final drafting.

Case #5: A neuropsychology trainee is completing a post-doctoral fellowship in a large medical center. She conducts a comprehensive evaluation of an outpatient child who was referred by a pediatric neurologist. The patient and her family are frightened and worried due to the recent onset of seizures and motor tics in the child. When the trainee meets with her supervisor to discuss the test results (that showed significant deficits), the supervisor dismisses the need for any type of in-person feedback. She says, "It's more important for you to give feedback to the neurologist. The kid's family won't understand a lot of this anyway and you don't want to be the one to give them bad news. Just mail them a copy and tell them that they can call you if they have questions."

These cases represent some examples of patients' and psychologists' experiences during a neuropsychological examination. In each case, there are the following common themes:

(1) The patient does not understand the nature of a neuropsychological examination and is confused as to the purpose, methods, and potential outcomes;
(2) Patients are often not informed of the results, except for final conclusions. This leads to even more confusion because the rationale for the conclusions is unclear;
(3) There is an aura of secrecy around the whole process.

Neuropsychological assessment procedures typically follow an "Information Gathering Model" of assessment. This will be discussed further in the next chapter, but suffice it to say that in an information-gathering model of assessment, the evaluator is a detached observer who administers a series of tests to a relatively passive and uninformed patient. *Uninformed* means that the patient is generally not privy to the nature of the tests or what they purport to measure. Second, the patient is not informed of the test results, either during the process itself or usually afterward. Thus, there is an aura of secrecy around the entire process, as if the examiner is using tools and techniques that are alien to the patient in order to initiate some kind of hidden agenda. The underlying assumption is that the patient may not understand or be able to handle the truth behind the nature of the testing process, and thus they are kept in the dark for their own good. Also, there seems to be a fear that if the patient knew about the nature of the testing methods, then this knowledge may lead them to bias the results in some manner.

This method of testing is very consistent with the medical model of assessment and treatment where the physician uses a series of tests in order to identify and isolate a disease process so that appropriate treatment can be initiated. In such a model, the patient's own thoughts, ideas, and judgments cannot be trusted because they lack the skill and objectivity to accurately contribute to sound diagnostic classification. An inherent part of this process is the assurance that the environment where the testing takes place is as sterile as possible. In a medical examiners office, sterility is important in order that no extraneous germs or diseases infiltrate the patient and confound the expression of symptoms lest diagnoses be rendered inaccurately. Similarly, in the neuropsychological examination, it is important that the environment be as cognitively sterile as possible in order that no extraneous influences confound the accurate depiction of the brain–behavior relationship. The ideal result is an accurate classification of the patient, based on a compendium of tests into a coherent and succinct cognitive profile. Historically, the purpose of developing such a profile was to identify specific brain–behavior relationships, but more recently, it is to assess and describe functional impairment in the hopes of providing guidance for care and possible remediation.

The advantages of an information-gathering/medical model of care can be likened to the advantages of a controlled clinical trial for researching a behavior therapy. In a controlled clinical trial using an experimental method, a researcher attempts to control as many extraneous variables, or noise, in order that the inherent processes that contribute to the effectiveness of a behavior therapy can be illuminated. The disadvantage of such an approach is that ecological validity is lost. Put simply, you cannot accurately depict how the behavior therapy will work in real life. Similarly, the information-gathering model allows you to examine the behavior of a patient under a structured and controlled situation, but you cannot definitely state how their functioning looks in real life. You lose the ability to observe the richness of human behavior and all its potentialities. What's more, in an effort to understand the person from a brain–behavioral perspective, one risks missing other important facets of the person that likely contribute to their cognitive and behavioral functioning. Missing these things may have consequences of developing conclusions that are incomplete and inaccurate and can lead to interventions that do not adequately address patient's needs. Consider the following example:

Ms. H was referred for testing by her primary care physician due to suffering some mild injuries after being hit by a car while bicycling. She hit her head (she was wearing a helmet) on the ground after falling from her bike, although her arms and body absorbed most of the force from the fall. Testing and evaluation from the emergency room and follow-up appointments revealed no evidence of a head or a brain injury. A few months after the accident, the patient began to experience memory problems and difficulty organizing at work. Neuropsychological testing was ordered, and the results indicated that the patient was performing well on nearly all tests of cognitive functioning, except for tests measuring attention, concentration, and working memory. In performing these tests, the evaluator noticed that the patient became particularly nervous and appeared to be trying to hold back tears. Supportive reassurance helped to some degree, but the patient performed below what would be expected for her age. The evaluator tested the limits on these tests and instructed the patient in relaxation and calming skills.

When alternative forms of attention and working memory tests were re-administered, the patient's performance improved significantly when she used the calming techniques. In exploring this further, the patient revealed a history of psychologically traumatic events. Clinical observation suggested that the patient's coping style was one of repression, which she admitted had been her style for many years. The recent accident triggered a flood of painful memories of past traumatic events that overwhelmed the patient's psychological resources and, as a result, her mind intermittently "shut down" in order to cope with the flood of emotions. Finally, her attention and concentration suffered, and her concomitant anxiety hindered her abilities even more. However, she was very intelligent and her other cognitive abilities were intact, which allowed her to cope and get through her days. The suggested diagnosis was post-traumatic stress disorder as opposed to what previously looked like a cognitive disorder due to post-concussion syndrome.

This example illustrates the potential consequences of blindly following the information-gathering medical model of assessment. Had the examiner not tested the limits and gathered more information about the patient's functioning, she might have been given an inaccurate diagnosis of an organic syndrome versus the more accurate diagnosis of an anxiety disorder. In this case, psychotherapy was recommended in addition to follow-up testing.

Another consequence of this approach is that patients who receive neuropsychological assessment services remain as peripheral observers of the process and have no opinion or impact on how the information is used for their benefit. Patients who feel this way may be less likely to express to the referring provider that their experience with the neuropsychological examination was positive. This may have a negative impact on the referring provider's perception of the psychologist, neuropsychological assessment, and the likelihood of wanting to use such services in the future. In contrast, patients who are empowered to be active participants in the neuropsychological assessment, through an open sharing of thoughts and impressions, being free to comment on the results and their applicability, and contributing to information that goes into a report, are likely to leave with a greater understanding of what neuropsychological assessment entails and how it can benefit them. Patients may then see the value of neuropsychological assessment, which translates into greater patient satisfaction and possible advocacy for the service.

This is the goal of collaborative therapeutic neuropsychological assessment (CTNA). The assessment is *collaborative* because it enlists the patient as an active participant who operates as a type of partner throughout the entire process of interviewing, testing, and feedback. The assessment is *therapeutic* because when patients are enlisted as active collaborators, they are more likely to take ownership of their own health care and work with professionals on making changes to improve their health and well-being.

In proposing CTNA methods, we are not suggesting that the information-gathering model of assessment be abandoned altogether. Certainly, there may be times when this format is appropriate. We suggest that the field of clinical neuropsychology consider broadening the perspective of assessment methods to incorporate a collaborative approach that is more in keeping with patient-centered care. A collaborative approach requires an open sharing of thoughts, ideas, information, and test data. Such a model challenges many assumptions inherent in the medical model and explored by Stanley Brodsky (1972).

Assumption 1: "We (the clinician) know best." This assumption implies that we as professionals, because of our training, education, and experience, have the knowledge the patient does not have, which therefore assumes that our opinions and interpretations are preeminent. The trap in this assumption is that we assume the patient does not have knowledge about themselves, which may be valuable in understanding their experience. In a collaborative approach, clinicians acknowledge that they have knowledge and experience that will be valuable for a patient, but that the patient may also have knowledge and experience that may be helpful in interpreting and understanding a cognitive profile. As a clinical supervisor once put it, "Psychologists are experts on human behavior; patients are experts on themselves. Both are necessary."

Assumption 2: "Patients are fragile." This implies that if patients were to know the results of tests or things that were said about them, this knowledge would be unbearable and distressing and may initiate psychological maladjustment. Certainly, there are times when clients may need to be protected from certain pieces of information, which requires sound clinical judgment. However, experience suggests that an open sharing can lead to patient empowerment because this arms them with knowledge. This assumption seems to stem from clinician's fear about causing patients harm or distress. As an example, in response to work in collaborative assessment, a colleague stated, "I don't want to be the one to tell someone they're brain damaged!" I wonder what makes this different from telling someone they are an alcoholic or a depressed or have diabetes or cancer? Giving patients information helps them understand the playing field and make realistic decisions about their lives. The important component is that such information must be given with *clinical skill and sensitivity*. This is the strength of collaborative assessment. The clinician can learn to share information in an open and sensitive way, which can empower the patient and not further impair them.

Assumption 3: "Patients will manipulate the results to their benefit." This assumption reflects a fear that once patients have the information, they will use it to their advantage to manipulate the doctor or the system. An example of this fear may be reflected in the following scenario.

During regular operations at an outpatient mental health clinic, a therapist was called to the front desk to help with an irate patient. This patient came into the clinic over two hours after the scheduled intake appointment and demanded to be seen and receive medication. The clinic policy was that no patient could receive medication the first day until they were scheduled and eventually evaluated by the psychiatrist. When this was explained to the patient, he glared at the therapist and proceeded to cite all that had ever been said about him in medical records he obtained. He stated that he was diagnosed with a severe mental illness, was tested to have various impairments, and was prescribed numerous different medications of which he knew their exact names, dosages, what they were used for, and even their generic names. At this point, he glared again at the therapist and stated if he did not get medication right now, he would leave this clinic and "blow his brains out."

This obviously extreme example is reflective of fears clinicians have about patients having too much information about themselves and then using it to manipulate others. Although these types of situations are always a risk, they tend to be infrequent, and often the type of patient who would behave in this manner would act the same way, no matter what type of information they received. Again, clinical judgment and knowing your patient's history and behavior patterns are important in helping you make such determinations. Most patients will use clinical information to understand themselves and empower them to manage their own health care.

Another example relates to the only known published study evaluating the effects of providing medical and neuropsychological information to traumatic brain injury patients (Pegg et al., 2005). In a personal communication with Dr. Pegg, he reported that patients who received this clinical information were much more informed about themselves and their condition. As a result, staff in the rehabilitation unit described them as more challenging because they constantly asked well-informed questions about their care now that they were armed with this new knowledge.

Another example relates to "The Case of Amy" (Gorske, 2008). Amy sought a neuropsychological evaluation to assess the post-operative effects of a grade IV glioblastoma. In my first meeting with Amy, she presented me with folders of medical records that she had obtained about her condition. Throughout our meeting, she asked many intelligent and often challenging questions about what we were going to do, the results, how they would be used, whether she could get copies, among others. This was a kind, gentle, and sensitive woman who was going to understand everything that was happening to her and what other people were saying they were going to do to her. Collaborative assessment challenges clinicians to step out of their expert role and meet the patient on an equal level. Most patients understand that professionals have knowledge and expertise patients don't have. Patients want professionals to use that knowledge for their benefit, but they don't want to be talked down to either. CTNA calls on the patient to give the clinician *permission* to use our knowledge and expertise for their benefit.

Another rationale is to contribute to the survival of clinical neuropsychology as a profession. As will be discussed in this chapter, the field of clinical neuropsychology, and one could argue psychology as a discipline, is suffering from an identity crisis due to many forces threatening its survival. Such forces include managed care; over-reliance on pharmacological interventions, thanks to aggressive marketing by pharmaceutical companies; and ongoing confusion in patients as to what differentiates psychology from psychiatry, social work, counselors, and coaches. Specific to clinical neuropsychology, patients often are confused as to the difference between a neuropsychologist, a neurologist, and a neuroscientist. The confusion as to what a clinical neuropsychologist does is further exacerbated by the advent of computerized testing, briefer and more user friendly cognitive examinations, and a trend where non-psychologists are using these tests to make clinical judgments without the use of psychologists.

One factor that determines whether a profession will grow and develop is its ability to examine and re-define itself over time. A profession will grow and thrive when its members look at the forces impacting its survival and then explore ways to adapt and change in order to face those forces. If a profession does not do this, it will become stagnant in its philosophies and methods and eventually become irrelevant to the needs of those who may seek out its services. The profession of psychology is no different in this regard. The study of forces that drive human behavior has undergone numerous transformations; unconscious psychic-driven forces, conditional social spheres leading to incongruence between the true and the ideal self, automatic negative thoughts, incorporation of parental introjects, reactions to social forces, a maladaptive wiring of neuronal connections, and an integration of all of these are only some of the theories developed that are thought to drive human behavior. Each of these ideas developed on the basis of new knowledge and, in some cases, the prevailing trend of thought at the time. Either way, ideas, knowledge, and discoveries led to adaptation and change of the professional psychology identity. The field of clinical neuropsychology is no different in that it has been forced to re-examine itself and contemplate the direction of change it wants to go. The difficulty lies in determining the direction of change. We will discuss three of the primary forces that have influenced the development of this identity crisis: technological advances, managed care, and patient-centered care.

Technological Advances

Originally, clinical neuropsychology's calling was to use assessment tools to aid in the identification of circumscribed brain lesions. This period in neuropsychology is referred to as the "Period of Neuropsychological Localization" (Ruff, 2003, p. 848). Prior to the 1970s, aside from neuropsychological tests, EEGs and x-rays were the primary tools for localizing brain damage. Neuropsychologists were important contributors in neurology, neurosurgery, and many other areas of medicine. Thanks to the work of pioneering neuropsychologists like Aleksandr Luria, Ward Halstead, Hans-Lukas Truber, Oliver Zangwill, Henry Hecaen, and many others, we have a wealth of knowledge on brain–behavior relationships.

Technology began to change the role of the neuropsychologist in patient care. The "Period of Neuropsychological Localization" drew to an end with the advent of more advanced radiological techniques such as PET, SPECT, CT, MRI, and fMRI. Though relatively crude and inefficient in the beginning, such neuroimaging techniques have become the cornerstone for diagnosing and localizing brain lesions. As more sophisticated techniques developed, and professionals became more adept at reading these images, the age of localization came to an end because now we could see where the damage was; we didn't need neuropsychological testing to pinpoint the brain lesion. The question arose, "What is neuropsychological testing needed for?" Ruff (2003) describes the next period as a "Period of Neurocognitive Evaluation." Spearheaded by Edith Kaplan and the Boston Process Approach, in this period, neuropsychological tests were used to describe various cognitive constructs such as verbal and visual learning and memory, verbal fluency, mental flexibility and set shifting, among many others. Because we now knew where the brain damage was, neuropsychologists were increasingly called upon to describe the cognitive and behavioral effects of damage. An examples of a referral questions that reflects this concept is as follows:

A middle-aged woman who suffered an infarct was referred to a neurologist. The pattern of deficits indicated an apraxia, suggesting left parietal damage. However, a review of the MRI revealed damage focalized in the insular. The neurologist wanted to know if there were any other deficits, not detected by standard neurological examination, that could be attributed to the location of the infarct.

Questions such as these shifted the focus of neuropsychological assessment from one of "where is the damage?" to "what does the damage mean for this patient's functioning?" Thus, in addition to describing neurocognitive constructs, neuropsychologists were asked to describe the functional implications of brain damage. Said in another way, neuropsychologists were placed in a position to defend the *relevancy* of their tests and results. Relevancy would become an important factor to consider, as the financial efficiency of neuropsychological assessment came under scrutiny with the influence of managed care.

Managed Mental Health Care

Although the concept of managed care goes back as far as the 1950s, the late 1980s and early 1990s saw the upcoming influence of managed care as a painful reality. Psychologists foresaw the influence of managed care as potentially damaging to the quality of patient care and as an increasing hole in their pockets. Psychologists appeared to react with anger and argued about the damage that managed care would cause. Many psychologists spent more time voicing their complaints rather than developing creative ways to cope with the new climate or examining the scope of their practices. Psychological and neuropsychological testing suffered under managed care. As a result, the frequency with which psychologists used testing as part of their services decreased dramatically (Groth-Marnat, 2000).

Groth-Marnat (1999a) identifies two main issues contributing to the decrease in test use by psychologists: the *increasing expansion of psychology's roles* and the *lack of clear-cut data on the financial efficacy and feasibility of testing*. The first issue, *increasing expansion of psychology's roles*, refers to the increasing presence of psychologists in new areas, such as industry forensics, administration and organizational development, evaluation research, and many others. In today's health-care climate, psychologists are increasingly forced to become creative in their career aspirations such that they might cobble together several different professional roles. One option is to take the route of developing fundable research ideas and engaging in grant writing. Although this can be challenging and exciting, the rigors of developing an idea, writing a grant, and then hoping that it is included in the increasingly limited funding stream can be a risky business for even the most seasoned researchers. Funding for the National Institute of Health has dropped significantly over the last 5–7 years, while the number of individuals competing for grant money has drastically increased. Another career option has been traditional private practice. While offering the possibility of increased freedom and potentially rewarding work, decreased reimbursements through managed care have left psychologists struggling to make ends meet. Thus, psychologists are increasingly called upon to become creative in their pursuits of meaningful, yet financially feasible, work.

The second issue, *the lack of clear-cut data on the effectiveness and feasibility of testing*, has historically been lacking, although this is beginning to change (see Meyer et al., 2001). Although testing has always been assumed to be a part of the psychologist's repertoire, in reality, there is very little information on the effectiveness of psychological testing in the enhancement of patient care. Additional criticisms included a lack of reliability and validity of testing in regard to patient outcomes and improvement in well-being (Groth-Marnat, 1999b). Essentially, health-care administrators, providers, and other funding bodies were asking two questions, "What good is testing?" and specifically, "What good is testing for improving patient outcomes in a reliable and financially feasible way?" These were the realities psychologists faced as managed care began approaching like a steamroller. However, administrators and providers weren't the only ones asking these questions. Patients increasingly demanded that psychologists utilize an assessment process that would accurately identify their needs, communicate their results in a meaningful and respectful way, and provide guidance in ways to use the test results for their benefit.

Patient-Centered Care

Over the last 30 years, patient-centered care in medicine has been an important development in efforts to improve patient health and wellness. The overarching philosophy of patient-centered care is defined by a collaboration between the patient and health-care provider in developing of treatment plans that address areas of importance to the patient, as well as those recommended by professionals. For health-care providers to collaborate with a patient, two conditions must be present. First, the provider must listen and empathize with the patient's experience. This serves to enlist patients as collaborators by giving them the message that they are heard and understood, and their thoughts and opinions valued. Second, providers must respect patient's thoughts and opinions and consider these in developing recommendations for care. Patient-centered care has many different definitions, yet some common dimensions have been proposed that are contrary to the biomedical model (Mead & Bower, 2000). First, illnesses are viewed from a biopsychosocial perspective. This means that there is less of an emphasis on reductionism and more focus on the multiple factors (e.g., biological, psychological, social, and environmental) that contribute to the development of an illness. Second, the patient is seen as a unique individual and therefore has a unique perspective on what an illness means for them and their lives. This calls for physicians to consider the interplay of the patient's unique perspective in the treatment of an illness. Third, patient centeredness promotes an egalitarian relationship between doctor and patient. In patient-centered care, the traditional view of the doctor as "all knowing" is replaced with a collaborative model of doctor–patient collaboration and cooperation. This challenges doctors to respect patient autonomy and enlists patients as active decision-makers in their own health care. A fourth principle reflects an emphasis on the therapeutic alliance between doctor and patient. A strong therapeutic alliance is characterized by doctor's empathy for the patient, a spirit of collaboration, and respect for the patient's autonomy. Finally, the principle of "doctor-as-person" reflects traits of humanness and warmth in the physician. More importantly, in patient-centered care, the doctor and the patient mutually influence each other. As opposed to being an objective, a detached observer in the consultation, the doctor brings in aspects of himself/herself as part of the practice (Mead & Bower, 2000).

An example of a non-patient-centered interaction might sound as follows:

Physician: Mr. Smith, I have the results from your physical. It looks as though you are about 60 pounds overweight with a BMI of 28. I would suggest you begin a diet as soon as possible. We will have our nurse refer you to a nutritionist in our office who will review your current diet and recommend a healthier diet to get you to a better weight.

Patient: Um, well, ok. But I'm not sure if I'm ready for something like that.

Physician: I know it's hard, but this is important. A high body mass index puts you at risk for many health problems like diabetes, heart conditions, and artheriosclorosis just to name a few. Here is the prescription, do you have any questions?

Patient: (Sighs) No I guess not.

An example of a more patient-centered interaction might look as follows:

Physician: Mr. Smith, I have the results of your physical. We can discuss any number of things but I'd like to know if you have anything in particular you are concerned about.

Patient: Well, I guess I was wondering about my cholesterol.

Physician: Certainly, the results of your test indicate your cholesterol level to be at 251. Do you understand what that means?

Patient: Well I understand that to be high. (Has an anxious look on his face.)

Physician: That's correct Mr. Smith. It looks as if this concerns you somewhat.

Patient: I am. Does this mean now I'm going to have to follow some strict diet?

Physician: Following a prescribed diet is certainly one thing we can help you with. However, perhaps you'd like to hear some options I've told other people and what's worked for them.

Patient: Oh yes, I would.

This second scenario is more consistent with a patient-centered communication style. In this scenario, the physician inquires about *patient* concerns, assesses patient reactions and his/her level of understanding, reflects an understanding of the patients' reactions to the information given, and offers to provide a menu of options for the patient to consider. Patient-centered collaboration has become an important focus for health care because there is evidence that such an approach enhances patient–physician communication, adherence to treatment recommendations, and improves health outcomes (Mead & Bower, 2002; Flach, McCoy, Vaughn, Ward, Bootsmiller, & Doebbeling, 2004; Zandbelt, Smets, Oort, Godfried, & de Haes, 2007). Problems encountered in these outcome studies include varying definitions of patient-centered care, different outcomes for different patient populations, and different ways of measuring patient-centered behavior. In essence, the patient-centered care ideology is more developed than patient-centered empirical knowledge (Bensing, 2000). Authors have begun to rectify this problem by developing and testing patient-centered behavior coding instruments in order to assess the essential factors that make patient-centered communication effective (Zandbelt, Smets, Oort, & de Haes, 2005). This research continues to develop and will likely become an important part of physician–patient interactions as well as education for medical students.

Increasingly, we all expect a greater amount of information about health and disease states in order to make informed decisions about our care and treatments. We all want professional and competent advice about ways to improve our health and well-being, yet we also want our individuality and autonomy to be respected so we are empowered to make health-care decisions that fit our needs and lifestyles. Patients who seek out, or are referred to, neuropsychology services are similar in regard to these needs.

Developing a Patient-Centered Orientation

Having the terms "patient-centered" and "neuropsychological testing" in the same phrase may seem like an oxymoron. A patient-centered orientation has been associated with humanistic psychology, Carl Rogers, and client-centered psychotherapy, while testing has generally been more closely associated with a medical model type of intervention (this will be covered in greater depth in Chapter 2). Testing has been seen as dehumanizing by most humanistic practitioners because of the emphasis on identifying and diagnosing discrete constructs that lead to intervention versus considering the person as a whole. Neuropsychological testing has been looked upon in the same vain and arguably to an even greater degree because of its roots in medicine, neuroscience, neurosurgery, and neurology. This viewpoint has led neuropsychological testing to be viewed in the same manner as a blood test, colonoscopy, or gynecological exam: a procedure that is probably necessary in order to develop an accurate diagnosis but is uncomfortable and dehumanizing in its methods.

However, the roots of neuropsychology are more consistent with a patient-centered philosophy than one might think. The precursors of contemporary neuropsychology did not have the advantage of modern technological assessment tools and techniques to accurately discern the connection between brain and behavior. They had to rely on the tools of the time, which primarily consisted of relatively crude brain wave measures but mostly good old-fashioned clinical observation and intuition. A most notable scientist/artist (the term artist is mine) was Aleksandr Romanovich Luria. Luria not only made brilliant observations about brain–behavior relationships, but also captured the phenomenology of the person. In his book, *The Man with a Shattered World*, Luria captures the essence of Zasetsky's struggles to recover from a bullet injury to the left parietal – occipital area. He ends the story with a concise, yet succinct, summary of Zasetsky's plight:

> Although we have come to the end of this story it has, in fact, no real end. The man still lives with his family...which, over the years, has grown into a much larger settlement....As in years past, he sits at his desk each morning working on his story, trying to express himself better, to describe the hope and despair that are part of his continuing struggle. His wound healed twenty-five years ago, but the formation of scar tissue has resulted in attacks. The damaged areas of the cerebral cortex could not be restored....He desperately wanted to wake from this terrible dream, to break through the hopelessness of mental stagnation, to find the world clear and comprehensible instead of having to grope for every word he uttered. But it was impossible.... So he

reverted to the past, for he could not understand why the world had become so peculiar, why war was necessary, or find any justification for what had happened to him. Twenty-five years before he had been a gifted young man with a promising future. Why did he have to lose his memory, forget all the knowledge he had acquired, become a hopeless invalid condemned to struggle for the rest of his life? This was simply beyond him....He continues to try to recover what was irretrievable, to make something comprehensible out of all the bits and pieces that remain of his life. He has returned to his story and is still working on it. It has no end. (Luria, 1972).

This synopsis portrays not only the struggles Zasetsky had while trying to recapture his lost cognition, but also the human struggle of regaining a loss of self that has disappeared. It is clear that the loss of cognitive function is not only a medical issue but also a deeply human and existential issue reflecting a loss of personhood.

Essentially, we hope to begin to draw a line between neuropsychological *testing* and neuropsychological *assessment*. In its basic form, *testing* is merely a process of using tests, tools, and techniques to quantify a patient's cognitive strengths, weaknesses, and limitations. This pattern of weaknesses might correspond to a particular diagnosis, or it may merely be descriptive. As Handler and Meyer (1998) pointed out, *assessment* is a complex clinical interaction between a patient, his or her test data, and a skilled psychologist. In neuropsychological *assessment*, test data are integrated with patient history, corroborating data, family information, personality factors, contextual circumstances, and medical information to create a picture of who a person *is* at a particular period of their life. Although neuropsychological testing is a complex technical enterprise, it is clinically simplistic and lacking in psychological richness. Neuropsychological assessment is clinically complex, psychologically deep, and personally meaningful to the patient and/or his or her family.

Defining a Person-Centered Orientation

A person-centered orientation in psychotherapy is consistent with a humanistic model of psychology that emphasizes the importance of the therapeutic relationship as an agent of healing and growth (see Rogers, 1942, 1951). Although there are different factors that contribute to the effectiveness of a psychotherapeutic encounter, such as positive client expectations, acquisition of new behaviors, and a sound theoretical framework, another set of factors includes such therapist behaviors as warmth, unconditional positive regard, and the development of a collaborative alliance (Wampold, 2001). These person-centered relationship factors are thought to contribute to a high percentage of variance in what makes psychotherapy effective. Stated simply, the creation of a warm, trusting, empathic, and collaborative relationship is the crux of a person-centered orientation, and these conditions are essential factors in what makes psychotherapy effective (Wampold, 2001).

The advantages of developing a more person-centered orientation in neuropsychological assessment include enhancing the quality of services and improving outcomes with regards to diagnostic clarity and treatment recommendations. Enhancing the quality of neuropsychological assessment services essentially means that the patient and referral sources are satisfied with the work that was done. In order for them to be satisfied, professional and competent service must be provided. However, patients are not only seeking expertise but also wish to be treated as active collaborators in their healthcare decisions. Patients wish to be informed about the nature of professional services, the provider's ability to provide them, how the results are determined and what are the implications for their health and well-being. A person-centered orientation respects the needs of patients to be active participants in the healthcare process. In the case of neuropsychological assessment, this means enlisting the patient as an active partner in each phase of the assessment process and in the communication of results.

One of the challenges in a neuropsychological assessment is to obtain maximum effort from the patient in order to elucidate their true cognitive capabilities. There are many factors that influence a patient's effort in neuropsychological testing, including energy level, mood, whether they've had adequate sleep and nutrition, medical conditions, medications, and many others. Another factor often overlooked is the quality of the relationship with the examiner. A non-collaborative relationship can potentially influence a patient's effort on test results. Examiners who are cold and distant may create an atmosphere of tension where the patient feels more like a lab rat responding to orders than a human being collaborating in an important encounter. Consider the following example of a patient who is discovering that their memory is not as strong as they previously thought. In this example, the patient was read the first story from the Wechsler Memory Scale–III, Logical Memory, and found that despite intense concentration, they remembered very little of the story.

> *Patient* (looking worried, eyes wide open): Oh my god! I can't believe this! That's a simple story; I shouldn't have any problem remembering it!
>
> *Examiner*: Ok, let's move on to the next task (begins to read instructions for the second Logical Memory story).
>
> *Patient* (looking at the examiner, almost with a pleading facial expression): This isn't funny! I can't believe I don't remember that!
>
> *Examiner*: Ok, well let's move on.
>
> *Patient* (eyes tearing): This is a problem. Geez! What am I going to do?
>
> *Examiner*: Let's try this next task, ok?
>
> *Patient* (slumps back in the chair): Fine, go on.

Now consider an alternative way this interaction might go.

> *Patient* (looking worried, eyes wide open): Oh my god! I can't believe this! That's a simple story; I shouldn't have any problem remembering it.

Examiner: You seem really worried about this.

Patient: Well yes, that was a short story. I tried real hard to keep it in my mind but once you stopped reading it just left!

Examiner: It just kind of disappeared on you, huh? That's got to be frustrating.

Patient (giggling nervously): Yeah.

Examiner: Ok, well look. I have another story for you and I'm going to ask you to do the same thing. Why don't you take a deep breath, do the best you can and let's see what happens.

Patient (pauses, closes their eyes, and takes a deep breath): Ok, I'm ready.

In this example, the examiner took a few moments to offer support and encouragement, which may have helped the patient muster the energy to try their best. In the first example, the patient was clearly nervous and despondent going into the second story. This may have affected their effort in the recall of the story and provided a false picture of their true abilities. When undergoing an assessment of any type, patients are usually anxious from the beginning because they have already sensed (or have been told) that they have changed in some way. The idea that one's brain may have changed through injury, disease, aging, or some other factor is very frightening for most patients, and they look for some kind of reassurance. Obviously we as examiners cannot give them false hopes or assurances, but we can create a safe and trusting environment where the patient feels an alliance and support.

A person-centered approach can help examiners arrive at a more definitive diagnosis by facilitating self-disclosure by the patient, which can lead to a greater understanding of the nature of cognitive processes. In traditional models of assessment, the evaluator is a detached observer who interacts as little with the patient as possible in order to develop a rather sterile conceptualization of the patient's abilities. The philosophy behind this approach is that if the examiner interacts with the patient, it might contaminate the results and therefore provide an erroneous assessment. However, another philosophy suggests that by interacting with the patient, the assessor may arrive at a more accurate conceptualization of the patient. Dr. Constance Fischer at Duquesne University in Pittsburgh, Pennsylvania, developed a method of psychological assessment called Collaborative Individualized Psychological Assessment (see Chapter 2 for a review). Her method emphasizes active patient involvement in the assessment process and an interactive style by the examiner. The examiner is free to deviate from standard protocol in order to test limits and hypotheses or question the patient as to their personal process in completing test items. This method is not unlike Aleksandr Luria's method of neuropsychological assessment. Luria would use procedures to develop initial hypotheses about a patient's cognitive and behavioral functioning and would freely interact with the patient in order to assess various facets of their behavioral repertoire. From these initial hypotheses, Luria would then administer another round of tests in order to confirm or disconfirm these hypotheses, thereby developing a more comprehensive picture of their abilities (see Chapter 2 for a more comprehensive description of Luria's methods). In the following example, a young woman, sought neuropsychological testing due to concerns of having a learning disorder that was affecting her college studies.

Barbara had never been identified or tested as having a learning problem throughout grade school, middle school, or high school and, in fact, was in accelerated classes although she was never formally identified as gifted. She described that her early school years were easy and that she never had to work very hard to get straight A's. In college, however, she struggled with different classes, particularly math classes and any class where she had to take tests under a time constraint. Her cognitive profile revealed above average to superior abilities in most areas of cognitive functioning. However, she performed below what might be expected on tests that included a time component. During one of the timed tests of achievement, the following behaviors were noted. She began to breathe faster, her shoulder's hunched, she gripped her pencil tightly, and her legs shuffled throughout the test. She periodically made nervous gestures such as wringing her hands, playing with her hair, and tapping the table. These gestures seemed to increase in intensity every time the examiner reminded her how much time she had left. Once the test was completed, the examiner reviewed her answers. The results indicated that she missed items she should have known well. The examiner reviewed these results with her, and she became frustrated because she knew the answers and couldn't understand how she missed them. The examiner discussed the patient's behaviors, thoughts, and feelings during the test. She disclosed that she was nervous because she was worried about getting them all right and feared the ramifications of failure if she didn't finish under the time constraint. The examiner suggested she try an alternate form of the test again, but this time the examiner guided her through some relaxation procedures and developing alternative thought processes that reframed her thoughts of failure. When she took the alternate form of the test, she was guided through the relaxation procedures and finished the test within the time frame and was able to accurately complete the problems. Through further discussion, it was discovered that she frequently experiences these types of nervous feelings and behaviors and as a result becomes distracted and unfocused. It was agreed that a diagnosis of anxiety, specifically test-related anxiety, was more accurate than a learning disorder.

This is an example where a process approach helped to formulate a more accurate depiction of the patient's struggles than simply relying on the numbers. By allowing Barbara to express her thoughts and feelings about a particular task, the examiner can learn what mental processes the patient uses, which help or hinder her performance. In this way, a person-centered approach can aid in formulating a more accurate diagnosis by using the patient's own experience as a guide. This type of approach is becoming an essential component in the fields of cognitive rehabilitation.

Patient-Centered Rehabilitation and Treatment

Over the last 20 years, cognitive rehabilitation of individuals with brain injuries has received more attention. This is due to literature showing that individuals with brain injuries, whether due to a traumatic event, stroke, disease, toxin, or some other neurological illness, often experience deficits in cognitive, behavioral, and general functional abilities and that cognitive rehabilitation is a valuable tool in helping brain-injured patients resume productive lives (Cicerone et al., 2005; Klonoff et al., 2006; Katz, Ashley, O'Shanick, & Conners, 2006). Thus, programs have been developed to meet the needs of brain-injured patients, and these programs have begun to evaluate the effectiveness of their methods in order to provide models of rehabilitation that can be replicated. Many of these programs follow a holistic model of rehabilitation where one of the key principles is to consider the patient's phenomenological viewpoint of the injury and rehabilitation process in order to enlist them as an active partner. This principle stems from increasing knowledge that enlisting active patient involvement is a key element in the success of a rehabilitation program.

One of the factors contributing to active patient involvement in a rehabilitation program is a solid and collaborative working alliance between the patient and the practitioner. The importance of a working alliance in successful psychotherapy has been well documented in the literature (Martin, Garske, & Davis, 2000). More recently, a positive working alliance has been identified as a key factor in helping patients change various health and mental health behaviors. In the field of addiction recovery, the standard of treatment for many years was the "confrontation of denial approach." This approach emphasized some specific principles: (1) heavy emphasis on acceptance of a problem, specifically a diagnosis, (2) emphasis on pathology, which reduces personal choice, judgment, and control, (3) a practitioner presents problems to the client in order to convince them to accept a diagnosis, (4) resistance is seen as denial, which is met with therapist confrontation, arguments, and correction, (5) treatment decisions are made by the therapist because the client is unable to make sound decisions due to being in denial (Miller & Rollnick, 1991, 2002). Over the last 20 years, this approach has been replaced by a motivational approach that emphasizes active patient empowerment, an empathic therapeutic relationship, and a trust in the patient to be an active partner and guide the treatment decision-making process. This approach has become the gold standard of addiction treatment and has demonstrated positive patient outcomes in multiple clinical trials (Hettema, Steele, & Miller, 2005).

In the field of cognitive rehabilitation, a similar process appears to be taking place. Practitioners and researchers are beginning to recognize the importance of developing a collaborative working alliance with rehabilitation patients due to evidence suggesting that such an alliance has a positive impact on outcomes. A collaborative working alliance is generally developed through a client-centered interpersonal style, one that respects patient's individuality and autonomy and empathizes with their individual perception of their situation (Schönberger, Humle, Zeeman, & Teasdale, 2006; Van den Broek, 2005).

Another patient-centered concept is an open sharing of diagnostic and clinical information. Whereas in the past, it was thought that certain clinical or diagnostic information should be hidden, a patient-centered philosophy calls for openness and willingness to dialogue with the patient about such information. The good news about this is that there is evidence to suggest that psychologists do regularly share such clinical information with patients. What remains unclear is whether this sharing of information is having a positive effect on patient care and outcomes.

Psychologists are Giving Feedback: A Survey of Feedback Practices

In order to know whether a model for providing neuropsychological test feedback would be a valuable tool, it first helps to know if this is standard practice among psychologists. Although there is ample information on the conduct of neuropsychological assessment interviews and test procedures, the provision of feedback has received little attention in the literature. This, however, appears to be in contrast to what is done in clinical practice where practitioners frequently refer to feedback sessions when discussing work with their patients. The question remains, how common a practice is it for psychologists to give in-person feedback?

To answer this question, we conducted an Internet survey. A full description of the survey and its results can be found at Smith, Wiggins, and Gorske (2007). We surveyed 3,217 members from the National Academy of Neuropsychology, International Neuropsychological Society, and the Society for Personality Assessment. Our return rate was 22%, which equals 719 participants. We surveyed their training and background including clinical experience, years of practice, work settings, and current assessment practice. Second, we asked about the types and frequency of tests used and finally feedback practices. The feedback questions consisted of a five-point Likert scale where participants were asked to rate the frequency with which different feedback practices had varying effects.

The results indicated that about 71% of those surveyed "usually or almost always" provide in-person feedback to their patients and that the majority of them (46%) spend about 50–60 minutes in a feedback session. Also, there was no difference between NAN, INS, and SPA participants in regard to the amount of time spent in feedback. Thus, the results suggest that in-person feedback is a frequent clinical undertaking with the majority of respondents spending at least a clinical "hour" providing test results. Given that providing feedback appears to be a frequent clinical endeavor, the next question is, what effect does providing feedback have on patients and/or family members?

To answer this question, we asked survey participants to rate the perceived effect of feedback on the patients and families they serve. Again, the results were overwhelmingly positive. Survey participants indicated that feedback sessions had the effect of usually or almost always facilitating an open dialogue (72%), helped patients understand their problems better (75%), were generally a positive experience for patients (75%), and that patients were generally satisfied with the feedback (76%). In addition, survey participants indicated that patients were usually or almost always active participants in the feedback process (68%), were more motivated to follow recommendations (52%), and that patients and/or family members felt better as a results of the feedback (67%).

So, in general, clinicians who provide feedback from neuropsychological tests perceive it as a positive endeavor with equally positive effects. One important limitation of this survey is obvious – it reflects clinician perception versus patient perception. This is an area that has yet to be fully researched. We found only a few studies that address consumer perception of neuropsychological assessment.

Bennett-Levy and colleagues (1994) evaluated consumer satisfaction with neuropsychological services by evaluating three primary procedural variables inherent in a neuropsychological evaluation: expectations and preparation for the assessment, the testing process itself, and discussion and feedback (Bennett-Levy et al., 1994). Using a survey based on interviews with patients, they found that over half of the patients' surveyed viewed the overall experience as positive (56%). In regard to patients receiving a discussion/feedback session, they found that 68% of respondents received feedback versus 32% who did not. Of those patients who received feedback, the majority found it to be useful (67%), helpful in learning about personal strengths (57%) and problem areas (67%), learning about what the results mean for everyday life (57%), and ways to get around problem areas (50%) (Bennett-Levy et al., 1994). Interestingly, 59% of respondents wanted more information than what they received versus 39% who felt the amount was adequate.

Bennett-Levy and colleagues' conclusions about the meaning of their data offer important insights into the role of feedback in the neuropsychological assessment process. They see the assessment process and the consequent feedback within the framework of patient-centered communication with medical providers. Two of these important insights include the following: nearly a third of respondents indicated that the feedback was not understandable and they did not remember it; the majority of respondents would have liked more feedback than they received (Bennett-Levy et al., 1994). It appears that an important component of neuropsychological test feedback for patients is that they can understand and integrate it in a way that they can remember and use the information. Second, that they want ample feedback in order to help understand what they are going through.

Donofrio, Piatt, Whelihan, and DiCarlo, (1999) evaluated consumer perceptions of neuropsychological test feedback. They assessed the perceptions of 60 patients who received one-hour feedback sessions following neuropsychological evaluation. They found that all patients found the sessions helpful (16.7%) or very helpful (83.3%) and that the recommendations were also helpful (21.7%) or very helpful (73.3%). An important component is that 92% of the patients reported that they would refer other people to the clinic as a result of their experience (Donofrio et al., 1999). Overall, their conclusions emphasized the importance of feedback in improving the quality of patient care with neuropsychological assessment.

To summarize, it appears that based on the limited literature, providing feedback from neuropsychological tests is frequently practiced by clinical psychologists and neuropsychologists and the effects of feedback are generally positive and likely to enhance the quality of patient care. Despite this knowledge, there is no model that establishes a "best practice" approach for conducting a feedback session from neuropsychological tests. Second, when psychologists say they conduct feedback sessions, it is unclear exactly what they are doing. Based on the Smith et al. (2007) study, about 71% of psychologists provide in-person feedback. Does that mean they are simply telling patients the results of the tests consistent with a traditional information-gathering approach? An unresolved issue is the nature of the feedback encounter. What is the feedback process, and what can happen during this process to make the session most helpful for patients? This issue is unclear because there is no best practice standard as to what constitutes a feedback session in general, and more specifically, what constitutes a *good* feedback session. CTNA methods provide a model of care for conducting a feedback session that adequately elucidates a methodology that is therapeutic for patients and increases their satisfaction with care.

A Proposed Model

We are proposing a model of CTNA as a patient-centered method for conducting an initial neuropsychological assessment interview and feedback session. We believe that developing such a model fills an important gap in neuropsychological assessment methods. The gap is the need to develop a more patient-centered neuropsychological assessment and feedback process that enlists patients as active collaborators and empowers them to take charge of their own cognitive health. We hope that doing so leads to greater patient satisfaction with neuropsychological assessment services, enhancing motivation to obtain such services, facilitating follow through with treatment and rehabilitation recommendations, and encouraging referral sources, other providers, and funding bodies to see CTNA as an important component of patient care.

Chapter 2
CTNA Conceptual Foundations: A Brief History of Psychological and Neuropsychological Assessment Feedback

In this chapter we will discuss the models that comprise the conceptual foundation of CTNA. CTNA's framework lies in the traditions of Therapeutic Assessment (TA) Models whose principles espouse a person-centered philosophy that views tests and test results as tools for understanding a patient's life and working to rewrite their life stories in a way that facilitates healing and growth. The methods for accomplishing this goal are based on recommendations for providing neuropsychological test feedback and the Motivational Interviewing principles for providing objective feedback in a person-centered manner. Motivational Interviewing principles will be discussed in Chapter 5.

Background of Neuropsychological Test Feedback

The literature is limited on the use of neuropsychological tests as therapeutic interventions or the development of a feedback process. What follows is a description of different authors' recommendations for providing feedback from the results of neuropsychological tests. This section will begin with a description of Aleksandr Romanovich Luria's Neuropsychological Investigation as a qualitative method for conducting neuropsychological examinations. This will be followed by recommendations in the literature for providing objective feedback from the results of neuropsychological tests.

Luria's Neuropsychological Investigation

Luria's Neuropsychological Investigation (LNI) is not a formal feedback method, but its components are highly consistent with a phenomenological analysis of patients' neuropsychological test results. LNI was a method developed by the Russian neuropsychologist Aleksandr Romanovich Luria for understanding syndromes of behavioral disturbance due to circumscribed brain lesions. A full review of the procedures is beyond the scope of this book, and the reader is referred to the comprehensive description provided by Anne Lise Christensen

T.T. Gorske, S.R. Smith, *Collaborative Therapeutic Neuropsychological Assessment*,
DOI: 10.1007/978-0-387-75426-0_2, © Springer Science+Business Media, LLC 2009

(1975/1984) or Luria's book (Luria, 1966). This section will be limited to a description of the qualitative methods used by Luria during a neuropsychological investigation.

Luria's method is a qualitative approach to examining patient functioning that requires variability and flexibility on the part of the investigator. Luria's examination method began with a preliminary conversation with the patient. This was considered essential in order to establish a positive, therapeutic atmosphere that elicited the patient's cooperation and emphasized a trusting, collaborative, problems-solving, and working relationship between the examiner and the patient. Luria would provide a series of brief standardized tests in order to develop hypotheses about the patient's functioning and would then conduct a more individualized neuropsychological assessment based on mental process defects discovered in the initial examination. A key feature of this examination was that it was flexible and interactive. Finally, the examination ended with a psychological conclusion that was shared with the patient (Christensen, 1975; Christensen & Caetano, 1999a). Luria discouraged the use of highly static and standardized methods of investigation. The current Luria Nebraska Neuropsychological Examination was developed by Charles Golden and colleagues and reflects more of a Western, quantitative approach to neuropsychological assessment that was rejected by Christensen and colleagues (Christensen, 1975; Christensen & Caetano, 1999a, 1999b).

Luria's methods were highly compatible with principles of Neuropsychological Rehabilitation. The qualitative and flexible nature of the method made it ideal for use as a psychotherapeutic approach (Christensen & Caetano, 1999a). Although not a formal feedback procedure, LNI used feedback to patients to enhance awareness about functional strengths and weaknesses and to ascertain patient responses to formulate diagnoses and treatment planning. Luria was influenced by Freud and the German humanistic philosophies. He wished to use scientific methods to understand individuals in context. Luria's interpretations of cognitive functioning would consider an individual's contextual framework for understanding a response to an inquiry. In order to elucidate these processes, Luria would take a hypothesis-testing approach, and the patient was initiated as an active collaborator in the hypothesis-testing process. As explained by Christensen and Caetano, "... the approach is phenomenological and interactive. There is a trusting therapeutic relationship between patient and Neuropsychologist ... an ongoing process of task modification, for example, giving the patient more time or explanations to complete a task, allowing the patient to copy tasks, or asking the patient to give his or her perception of the task ... so as constantly to provide feedback about the unique characteristics of the patient's strengths and deficits .... Luria would comment, asking questions and discussing issues in a highly involved manner such that the patient was included ... supported ... and given a sense of importance." (Christensen & Caetano, 1996).

Luria's method, although not a formal feedback procedure, contained elements identified by previous authors as important for providing information from the results of psychological tests. These include an emphasis on a collaborative therapeutic relationship; an open and flexible dialogue with the patient, which includes eliciting and sharing information from the results of the examination; a qualitative analysis that considers patient's individual contexts as influencing their performance; and a general patient-centered atmosphere where the patient is empowered as an active participant whose perceptions and opinions are valued and are, in fact, considered essential information in the final psychological conclusion. The next section will review the literature that has developed a conceptual framework for providing feedback from neuropsychological tests.

Recommendations for Giving Neuropsychological Test Feedback

Feedback from neuropsychological assessments has been thought of as optional and given limited consideration in the literature despite ethical obligations to fully inform patients about the nature and results of psychological tests and evidence to suggest that patients find such feedback useful, meaningful, and therapeutic (Gass & Brown, 1992; Pope, 1992; Armengol, Kaplan, & Moes, 2001). Feedback is important because it provides useful information about cognitive strengths and weaknesses and helps in the development of applicable interventions to enhance functional performance (Crosson, 2000). There is evidence that consumers find neuropsychological test feedback useful in identifying strengths and weaknesses and they apply it to everyday life concerns, which may be helpful in resolving life problems (Bennett-Levy, Klein-Boonschate, Batchelor, McCarter, & Walton, 1994). There is no agreed-upon conceptual framework for providing feedback from neuropsychological tests, although there are recommendations. Gass and Brown suggest that neuropsychological test feedback is an important intervention in and of itself with brain-injured patients, and they recommend a methodology for providing feedback from neuropsychological test data that is understandable, useful, and relevant (Gass & Brown, 1992). The methodology is summarized as follows: (1) review the purpose of testing in plain, simple language; (2) describe the tests as "behavior samples" that reflect domains of daily functioning; (3) explain test results in terms of domains of functioning and behavior; (4) summarize results in terms of strengths and weaknesses; (5) address any pertinent diagnostic issues; and (6) make appropriate recommendations (Gass & Brown, 1992, pp. 274–276).

There are no known empirically based studies assessing the effects of neuropsychological test feedback on variables related to treatment success with patients. Malla and colleagues used case studies to demonstrate the utility of neuropsychological test feedback in developing vocational rehabilitation plans for people diagnosed with a psychotic disorder (Malla et al., 1997). Allen and colleagues discussed the applicability of a process approach for neuropsychological assessment and feedback in order to provide psychiatric patients and their families information about deficits related to possible brain dysfunction

(Allen et al., 1986). These studies advocate for an informed neuropsychological assessment and feedback process that involves a "diagnostic partnership" with patients in order to provide accurate, in-depth information about cognitive performance that enhances patients' understanding of their functioning and develops realistic and applicable treatment goals (Allen et al., 1986; Gass & Brown, 1992; Malla et al., 1997).

Psychological Testing as a Therapeutic Intervention

Psychological testing has historically been looked upon with disdain, especially by humanistic practitioners, because testing was seen as a dehumanizing endeavor where the patient is viewed as an "object" to be observed and reduced to categories, traits, and diagnoses (Dana & Leech, 1974). Traditionally, psychological testing was conducted in a "top down" manner, with the evaluator providing a series of tests to a passive patient. The patient followed the examiners' instructions, completed the tests as required, and then had little input on the results, report, or decisions made from the results. This method of psychological testing was thought to stem from the medical model and psychometric traditions, where disease states are reduced to the most finite and measurable characteristics in order to contain, control, and treat. Just as the physician used laboratory tests or x-rays to concisely target the disease, psychological tests were seen as methods for reducing and concisely defining the mental disease process in order that it could be diagnosed and effectively treated through available methods. Dana and Leech trace the background of this philosophy to classical Newtonian thought where the external environment is considered separate from human beings' subjective experience and thus can only be known through objective observation. The fallout of this philosophical assumption was the dehumanizing of individual subjective experience and the objectification of humankind (Dana & Leech, 1974). Psychological testing was seen as a tool of this dehumanizing process.

This trend began to change with the development of models of psychological testing that emphasized patients' subjective experience and elicited their collaboration in the testing process. The advent of nondirective counseling methods (Rogers, 1942, 1951) changed the counseling emphasis from one of identifying unconscious forces that explain psychopathology to the creation of a trusting therapeutic environment where patients can feel safe to relinquish defenses and learn about themselves and their actualizing potentials. Some psychologists began to see how the use of psychological tests, administered under the conditions set forth by Rogers and other humanistic philosophers, can facilitate the development of self-knowledge, provided that the tests are used to *serve the needs of the patient* (Cronbach, 1949). These authors began to develop methods for using psychological tests as therapeutic interventions.

The use of psychological tests in psychotherapy emphasized performance-based (i.e., projective) testing methods and also frequently used self-report, intelligence, and cognitive tests (Aronow & Reznikoff, 1971; Bellack, Pasquarelli, & Braverman, 1949; Berg, 1985; Harrower, 1956; Luborsky, 1953; Mosak & Gushurst, 1972). Different authors have described the use of psychological tests in the psychotherapy encounter. Cronbach (1949) describes the use of tests in nondirective counseling only when the patient is ready or asks for such information. In describing the approach of Bordin, Cronbach emphasizes the empowerment of the patient who chooses what tests can be administered in order to answer questions that are important to them. Thus, the patient becomes the initiator of the testing process and is thereby responsible for the information they want to know about themselves. Another method is the provision of objective, graphical information about a patient's score in relation to others who have taken the test. Cronbach de-emphasizes the professional opinion of the psychologist and instead focuses on the provision of objective information that allows the patient to decide the meaning of the test results for their own lives. Instead of rendering a professional judgment as to what the test results mean, the evaluator would provide objective information about where a patient's test score falls within a plot or graph and what this score might mean in relation to a patient's question. The evaluator would then allow the patient to share thoughts and reactions and offer their own interpretation of what the test results mean for their lives. In regard to personality tests, Cronbach cites Bixler's opinion that the tests should be used to help the patient reflect on their feelings and to expand their understanding of themselves, versus using the tests as a way to diagnose or categorize a neurosis or a pathology. Additionally, Cronbach emphasizes that patients must be allowed to reject the interpretation of tests and that examiners should not become defensive or justify their results in order that patients feel free to openly and honestly examine themselves (Cronbach, 1949).

Molly Harrower (1956) developed a method for using patients' responses from performance-based tests as a way to develop insight and enhance the therapeutic process, which she termed "Projective Counseling Technique" (Harrower, 1956). The essence of the therapy is to elicit patient responses to clarify conflicts, confront the patient with their responses, and initiate a psychological reeducation process. The methods for her counseling technique are not well defined; however, some concepts can be deduced from her descriptions. The test interpretations are designed to facilitate patient insight, to develop ego integration and psychological adjustment, consistent with classic psychoanalytic theory. Harrower describes the use of test responses in much the same way as dream analysis (Wolff, 1956). Her methods could be considered primarily nondirective in that she would allow the patient to freely associate their projections and may even encourage the patient to provide their own interpretation, with the clinician providing guidance and suggestions.

Berg (1984) illustrated a model for a more flexible psychological testing process that considers the patient's interpersonal behavior as information for understanding test responses. His "Transactional Model" of the testing process emphasized a collaborative relationship between the examiner and the patient, which served to create a "psychological map" of the patient. Berg further developed a feedback process in which the examiner may comment on the patient's behavior during testing, all of which contributes to the collaborative endeavor. The elements of the feedback process include the following: (1) using language understandable to the patient; (2) gradually presenting psychological insights so as not to overwhelm the patient; and (3) providing brief information that is most useful, applicable, and relevant to the patient, the diagnostic process, and treatment recommendations (Berg, 1984). In addition, Berg emphasizes providing initial feedback that is within the realm of the patient's understanding and then gradually working toward deeper, unknown insights. This is consistent with Stephen Finn's perception that patients more readily hear information consistent with their own self-perception before they are ready to hear insights that are discrepant from their self-concept (Stephen Finn, 2007, personal communication). A fourth point relates to patient resistance. An examiner should use methods that lower resistance and foster collaboration, such as empathic evaluation, so that the patient may feel secure and free to continue commenting on the test material. Berg emphasizes that in reviewing the feedback at the end of testing, observations shared should have been mutually created by the examiner and the patient. In this way, the patient is an active collaborator in developing the assessment, feedback, and subsequent treatment recommendations.

Collaborative Individualized Assessment

Constance Fischer expanded on the view of psychology as a human-science endeavor by applying existential frameworks to psychological assessment. She posited an alternative to the deterministic "man-as-object" medical viewpoint in favor of a more collaborative "man-as-co-constitutor" of experience (Fischer, 1970). The psychological evaluation is one where the psychologist and patient work together and openly dialogue about the testing process. As collaborators, they mutually share findings and impressions, and the patient's experience and responses to the testing are understood in context of their life. Test results are shared in an open manner with the psychologist using down-to-earth terms, and the patient is free to openly dialogue about the interpretations provided (Fischer, 1970, 1994). This method is a change from traditional models that emphasize secrecy in psychological testing (Fischer, 1972). Collaborative Individualized Assessment (CIA) is based on phenomenological models of psychology that seek to understand a patients experience in the world as it is lived existentially, behaviorally, and reflectively (Fischer, 1979). In CIA, the assessor works collaboratively to understand a patient's unique worldview as it relates to the purpose of the assessment. Test scores, categories, and classifications are tools that serve to develop an understanding of the patient's life events.

CIA is conceived as a blend of the art and science of psychology into a "human science psychology" (Fischer, 2003), where the goal is to recognize human characteristics not easily captured by naturalistic science, yet remaining true to psychology as a scientific discipline. To accomplish this, a number of principles guide CIA. First, the assessor and patient *collaborate* in the assessment process. The patient is not a passive recipient of the assessors testing methods but is an active facilitator of the process and is thus empowered to share thoughts and ideas about the course of the assessment. Second, the patient's experiences and testing results are understood in the *context* of life events. The patient is not compartmentalized into simplistic categories, traits, or diagnostic constructs but is viewed as influencing and being influenced by the world in which they live. In CIA, the evaluator may *intervene* in the assessment process by deviating from standardized procedures in order to open the patient's experiential world and test alternative responses or reactions to the assessment. An assessor will use varieties of therapeutic dialogue to encourage deeper communication and openness by the patient, thereby more fully *describing* the patient's phenomenological world. Finally, patient's experiences are viewed in a *holistic* manner, where individual *complexity* and *ambiguity* are respected and there is no need to reduce experience to a series of traits, constructs, or other categorical systems (Fischer, 1979, 1994, 2000). CIA views the patient as a being "in process," with the testing activity serving as a microcosm of the individual's phenomenological world where the person becomes an active processor and creator of where they are and where they want to be (Fischer, 1979, 1994).

Therapeutic Assessment

TA shares many principles with CIA, and in fact, they have mutually influenced each other (Finn, 2007). In TA, psychological assessment is used as a therapeutic intervention. Its methods are strongly rooted in humanistic psychology, although this was not the primary philosophical basis (Finn & Tonsager, 2002). In TA, the tester is an active participant and the psychological assessment is an opportunity to facilitate rapport. Testers work collaboratively to develop empathic understanding with patients, openly dialogue about patient's responses to test stimuli, use the testing process to apply results to problems of daily living while exploring new ways of thinking and feeling, and pay attention to the interpersonal process to open further dialogue (Finn, 1996b; Finn & Tonsager, 1997; Finn, 2003).

TA uses the MMPI-2 in addition to performance-based tests, such as the Rorschach, and semi-structured psychosocial measures (Finn, 1996a, 2003; Finn & Kamphuis, 2006). There is empirical support for the utility of TA with college students. In one study, students seeking psychological services at university counseling centers were randomly assigned to receive feedback from the results of the MMPI-2 or clinician attention only. Results suggested that those who received feedback on their test performance reported increased self-esteem, decreases in symptomatic distress, and more hopefulness about improving their problems (Finn & Tonsager, 1992; Newman & Greenway, 1997). A case study illustrating the effects of TA with a man previously diagnosed with attention-deficit disorder showed how TA can be used as a professional consultation tool to explore a patient's life and struggles more deeply. This consultation model resulted in diagnostic clarification and direction in therapy as well. The result was that the patient was able to more fully understand and eventually change his "life story" (Finn, 2003). This case study illuminates the importance of a collaborative process where the term "feedback session" is actually a misnomer. A "feedback session" is a unidirectional approach where information is imparted from assessor to patient in a passive method. In the TA approach, the tester and the patient collaborate to apply and possibly rewrite patients' life stories (Finn, 2003). TA methods have expanded for use with different patient groups including those diagnosed with an eating disorder, borderline personality disorder, adult outpatients, severely emotionally disturbed children and their families, and executives being assessed for promotion (Finn & Martin, 1997; Michel, 2002; Finn, 2003; Finn & Kamphuis, 2006; Tharinger, Finn, Wilkinson, & Schaber, 2007; Fischer & Finn, 2008).

Summary of Psychological Testing as a Therapeutic Intervention

The use of psychological tests in the therapy encounter has a moderately rich history that has not broken into the mainstream of psychology. As a general framework, psychological testing methods merged with humanistic and existential principles. Thus, some common methodologies can be elucidated. First, testing is a collaborative endeavor with the psychologist and patient working together in the examination. Second, there is an open dialogue between the patient and the psychologist about the testing procedures and results so that the patient is an active participant in developing their own psychological profile. Third, there is a deviation from standard procedures or procedures are modified in order to elucidate aspects of the patient's psychological life not captured through standardized methods. Fourth, there is an open sharing of results. Patients are not kept in the dark about the test results but, in fact, may be co-interpreters of the information elicited from the tests. As such, the patient is empowered to agree or disagree with the results and to be an active creator of their own psychological life. Finally, diagnoses, norms, labels, and other constructs are used as tools to further understand the patient in context, as a whole person. Patient's psychological worlds are not reduced to traits or disease states, but these constructs contribute to an overall understanding of the individual. These principles are included in the CTNA, and their application will be explained further in the section on CTNA methods.

Contemporary Applications of Therapeutic Assessment and Neuropsychology

Therapeutic Neuropsychological Assessment (Gorske, 2008)

Therapeutic Neuropsychological Assessment (TNA) refers to a clinician's use of neuropsychological test results as a treatment method. The goal of the treatment is to facilitate change, healing, and growth with a patient who is suffering from some type of psychological condition. If there is no intention to treat, heal, or facilitate change, then the intervention is not therapeutic. For example, the goal of Collaborative Neuropsychological Assessment (CNA) developed by Dr. Steven Smith is to initiate the patient as a co-interpreter of neuropsychological test results. The goal is not to provide treatment but to enhance collaboration. One could argue that the collaborative nature is inherently therapeutic; however, this is not the primary goal. The goal of TNA, however, is to provide a treatment, hence the term therapeutic.

The Neuropsychological Assessment Feedback Intervention (NAFI) is a form of TNA developed as a brief intervention designed to enhance motivation for treatment adherence that involves the use of a semi-structured personalized feedback report. Any clinician who provides information from neuropsychological test results as a form of treatment conducts TNA. However, the use of the personal feedback report as a treatment entry intervention is what separates the NAFI from TNA. Although this may seem like semantics, it is important to provide this distinction for clarity. Essentially, the NAFI is more structured than TNA. TNA represents the heart or spirit of what the NAFI is trying to accomplish. NAFI is a brief treatment entry intervention that provides information about cognitive strengths and weaknesses and about how these cognitive strengths and weaknesses relate to important life problems patients may be experiencing. NAFI is not an educational intervention where a clinician provides information to passive patients in a "top down" manner. Patients are enlisted as active collaborators and are free to comment on the testing process and to discuss how the test results apply to their daily lives, they and are encouraged to share thoughts and reactions and agree or disagree with the information. The testing and feedback process is likely to be perceived as a therapeutic experience that uses the "tools" of neuropsychological testing to facilitate change, healing, and growth. Therefore, the clinician who conducts a NAFI session must have good clinical skills in developing a safe, empathic, and nonjudgmental therapeutic environment. NAFI uses the tools of Motivational Interviewing for developing therapeutic rapport, eliciting active patient collaboration, and lowering resistance that may be elicited from hearing test results.

The NAFI began development in 1999/2000 while Dr. Gorske was in postgraduate training at Western Psychiatric Institute and Clinic in a joint Addiction Medicine Services/Clinical Neuropsychology fellowship. For his post-doctoral experience, Dr. Gorske provided neuropsychological testing to patients diagnosed with a dual disorder (psychiatric and substance use disorder) in the Addiction Medicine Services Intensive Partial Hospital Program, a specialized group program serving dual-disorder patients. Dr. Gorske conducted and interpreted the test results under the supervision of Dr. Christopher Ryan, an internationally known neuropsychologist who, with the late Dr. Nelson Butters, studied cognitive factors in patients with alcoholism. The dual-diagnosis group was chosen for testing because there is very little information in the research literature on cognitive factors related to dual-diagnosis patients.

Earlier research on cognitive dysfunction associated with dual disorders focused primarily on schizophrenia with comorbid alcohol or cocaine use. Studies were inconclusive because they failed to determine that dual-diagnosed patients were more impaired than schizophrenic patients alone (Addington & Addington, 1997; Nixon, Hallford, & Tivis, 1996). Both schizophrenia and alcohol abuse disorders, independently, have similar impairments in abstract thinking and higher level reasoning skills, selective attention deficits, similar abnormal electrophysiological findings (such as reduced P300 amplitude reflecting disordered attentional processes), information-processing deficits, and memory deficits (Tracy, Josiassen, & Bellack, 1995). Studies that did find increased impairment in dual disorders reported deficits in learning and memory, abstraction ability, social comprehension, and verbal auditory perception (Serper, Bergman, & Copersino, 2000; Allen, Goldstein, & Aldarondo, 1999). The few studies conducted on cognitive functioning in non-psychotic dual-disorder patients indicate deficits in general intellectual functioning, problem solving, abstraction, verbal and visual memory, attention, calculation, comprehension, and visuospatial ability (Blume, Davis, & Schmaling, 1999; Carpenter & Hittner, 1997; Meek, Clark, & Solana, 1989).

After completing a testing session, the patients began to ask Dr. Gorske if they could receive feedback about the test results. Dr. Gorske and Dr. Ryan felt it was important to provide the information in a format that was clear and understandable to patients so they could be applied to their lives and problems related to their dual diagnosis. However, there was no agreed-upon conceptual framework for providing neuropsychological test feedback.

As part of his postdoctoral work, Dr. Gorske worked as research clinician and was trained to provide a specialized Motivational Interviewing intervention developed for a study funded by the National Institute on Drug Abuse for patients diagnosed with cocaine dependence and depression, led by Dr. Dennis Daley, one of the forerunners of research and treatment methods for dual-diagnosis patients. Part of the intervention included the use of a personalized feedback report similar to that used in the multisite Project MATCH studies (Miller, Zweben, DiClemente, & Rychtarik, 1992). The feedback report provided patients with objective information about the severity of their drug use, psychosocial impairment, diagnosis, and other personal information. However, the information from the feedback report did not seem to offer any new insight that was effective in motivating patients to make changes in their behavior. However, it was believed that the information from the neuropsychological tests might be useful to patients in providing relevant and applicable information about their cognitive and behavioral functioning, hence the idea to develop a personal feedback report based solely on neuropsychological test results.

The initial feedback report was three pages long and included basic information about neuropsychology and neuropsychological assessment and a brief description of patient's performance on individual tests. Patients who were tested were then given feedback from their neuropsychological test results. Anecdotal observations suggested that the patients were very pleased about the neuropsychological test feedback process. It appeared to enhance self-disclosure, and they began to talk about life areas they were concerned about, which the testing process seemed to elicit. They saw the applicability of the tests and the skills assessed to their daily lives. Most patients had some areas of cognitive compromise, either due to drug use or psychiatric illness, and they began to inquire about ways to improve their cognitive abilities so they could begin to lead more productive and fulfilling lives. From these promising observations, a more formal study of the NAFI began. Through funding from the Western Psychiatric Institute and Clinic Mental Health Intervention Research Center (MHIRC), Dr. Gorske gathered some preliminary data on the effectiveness of the NAFI in motivating patients to adhere to the Dual-Diagnosis Partial Hospital Program. In addition, data was gathered on patient satisfaction with the NAFI and that feedback was used to continually develop and crystallize NAFI methods. This preliminary data indicated positive outcomes that were compelling enough to obtain funding from the National Institute on Drug Abuse to conduct a more formal pilot study on "The Effects of Cognitive Test Feedback on Patient Adherence" (DA017273-01A1).

Pilot Study Results

A total of 30 patients were recruited for the study. The majority were women ($n = 18$, 60%) and Caucasian ($n = 23$, 77%), with the remaining patients being African American. The primary DSM-IV Axis I diagnosis, for substance use disorders, was alcohol dependence (27%) followed by cocaine dependence (7%). The most frequent Axis I mental health diagnosis was depressive disorder not otherwise specified (43%), followed by major depression (10%). The average age of patients was 38, with a mean education level of 2 years of college.

After patients agreed to enter the study and signed the appropriate consent forms, they received a small battery of neuropsychological tests. Afterward, the patients were randomly assigned to the NAFI feedback session or the treatment as usual (TAU) session, which included an orientation to the Dual-Diagnosis Partial Hospital Program at the Western Psychiatric Institute and Clinic Addition Medicine Services and a brief session emphasizing the importance of 12-step meetings and following the 12-step approach to treatment. The NAFI session was administered either by Dr. Gorske or by a trained research clinician. The

TAU session was administered either by Dr. Gorske or by a partial hospital staff member.

Two patients did not follow up after receiving the neuropsychological assessments, so they were not included in the adherence data. The results indicate that patients who received the NAFI session attended about 71% of the required group days versus the TAU group that attended 48% of the required group days. This difference was significant ($t = 2.139, p = 0.042$), with a moderately large effect size (bias corrected Cohen's $d = 0.78$, standard error $= 0.39$, 95% confidence interval $= 0.02 - 1.55$). A graphical illustration is presented below (Fig. 2.1).

In addition, both groups showed a decrease in their alcohol and drug use, although these differences were not statistically significant.

The patients' personal responses to the intervention were overwhelmingly positive. In order to assess this, a patient feedback form was administered following completion of the NAFI session. Comments made by patients included the following:

- "The assessment was helpful to me. I learned a lot about myself … I would have done it without being paid."
- "Allowed me to see why I may be reluctant to participate in groups."
- "Helped me narrow in on specific steps I need to take with my therapist re: depression and addiction. Identified a couple things we can work on."
- "I am so pleased that I participated in the study. It was right on. The clinician allowed me to share during the process, which really assisted with my overall understanding of the feedback."

This is the only known study that examines the impact of neuropsychological assessment feedback on patient treatment adherence rates. The results are

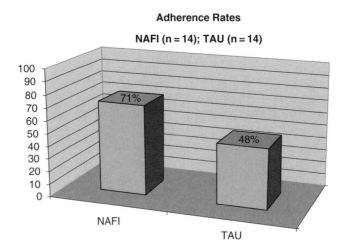

Fig. 2.1. Unpublished results from the NIDA study Effects of Cognitive Test Feedback on Patient Adherence

promising that such an intervention may be helpful in increasing patient satisfaction and improving attendance in formal treatment programs, especially with a challenging and traditionally treatment non-adherent patient group such as those with a dual diagnosis.

The obvious limitations of the study are that it contains a small and relatively homogenous patient sample. Additionally, the multitude of factors that may have contributed to patient adherence were not analyzed – one rather frustrating limitation related to the nature of the intervention itself. The NAFI was designed as a treatment entry intervention where patients receive a 1-hour session at the beginning of formal treatment. Afterward, they are sent to a traditional 12-step group program that emphasizes a more psychoeducationally based "confrontation of denial approach." Thus, it is possible that the patient-centered, individualized treatment experiences and recommendations were lost following the initial intervention. This could have impacted adherence rates and substance use outcomes. Future work may want to consider fashioning the treatment entry intervention and follow-up care so that they bridge similar theoretical frameworks.

Despite these limitations, the NAFI study is the first to examine a neuropsychological assessment feedback intervention and its affects on patient outcomes. The results appear to be promising enough to warrant examining such an intervention further and continually developing the framework of the model so that it can be used and adapted for other settings and patient populations.

Collaborative Neuropsychological Assessment

CNA was developed by Dr. Steven Smith from the Psychology Assessment Center at U.C. Santa Barbara. CNA was developed to bridge the gap between clinical neuropsychological assessment, interpretation of test results, and the provision of recommendations to patients and families. Unlike the NAFI, CNA was concerned not only with feedback but also with the overall clinical approach of neuropsychologists. This includes a focus on alliance building during interviews and testing sessions. CNA is based on TA research as well as psychotherapy process and therapeutic alliance work. In addition, CNA has a great deal of overlap with Gorske's TNA, and the two models have mutually influenced each other.

The three primary goals of CNA are as follows: (1) to provide answers to both the patient's questions and those of the referring professional; (2) to help the patient feel understood, and listened to by the clinician; (3) to provide the patient with a personal narrative-changing experience that will lead to greater insight, personal growth, acceptance, and/or responsibility. It is assumed that by working with the patient in a collaborative manner and attending to their needs, wishes, and emotional experiences, the results of the assessment will be more useful, powerful, and transformative. Given the centrality of the alliance in predicting treatment outcome in psychotherapy (Horvath & Symonds, 1991; Martin, Garske, & Davis, 2000), it is expected that the CNA approach will improve the alliance between the patient and the clinician, resulting in better test performance and greater follow-through with recommendations.

CNA is a patient-centered approach that views the patient as the most important informant in the assessment dialogue. This approach is appropriate primarily for patients without the most serious cognitive injuries or dementing conditions that might reduce the extent to which they can fully engage in the process. The clinical stance of CNA is to be open and accepting, interested, and concerned. The clinician works to seek answers to the patient's (or patient's family) specific questions so that the patient can have a greater understanding of themselves, their cognitive difficulties, and their day-to-day lives. CNA recognizes that the patient's difficulties have an emotional impact, causing distress, anger, and depression. Last, CNA recognizes that the most powerful assessment intervention is the feedback session, where assessors and patients can work together to understand the relationship between test findings and the patient's life struggles. The process of CNA proceeds in the following manner:

The initial interview: The goal of the initial interview is to understand the patient's symptoms and also the patient's emotional experience of those symptoms. This reflects the holistic viewpoint of CNA in understanding patient symptoms and individual perceptions, which are believed to be essential in understanding the nature of an illness or injury. There are four main components of the initial interview: understanding the problem, the patient's experience of the problem, the patient's wishes or fantasies about how the evaluation will help, and a socialization to the assessment process. Once the initial interview is complete, the testing proceeds according to standard procedures and administration guidelines. It is important to check the patient's clinical status as testing proceeds for fatigue, motivation, hunger, or any other factors that may contribute to quality of performance.

The feedback session: The primary goals in a CNA feedback session are to relay information to the patient regarding their performance on the tests and to relate this information to real-world difficulties that may compromise their cognitive and behavioral functioning. The outline for the CNA feedback session shares common methods with Ackerman, Hilsenroth, Baity, and Blagys (2000) and Hilsenroth, Peters, and Ackerman (2004) as well as the NAFI.

The method for conducting the session begins with the clinician asking the patient their fantasy about what they see as their strengths and later their weaknesses. The feedback begins with more global strengths and weaknesses (e.g., verbal and nonverbal processing) and moves to more specific skills (e.g., immediate sensory attention, semantic fluency). The key skills are to relay the information in layman's terms, free of jargon, and then to relate the information to patient's real-world functional concerns. Following feedback about strengths and weaknesses, a brief summary is given regarding the main points discussed.

Finally, the clinician provides a review summary of the key themes identified in each section of the feedback session. In addition, the clinician may present any diagnostic or other important mental health issues that would be important for the patient to know. The summary concludes with a review of patient questions, potential responses to those questions, and recommendations for further care or treatment. As is appropriate, the clinician will provide a list of resources that may be helpful for meeting the recommendations given.

The Neuropsychology Case Conference

The Neuropsychology Case Conference (NCC) model developed out of the Neuropsychology Program at Windsor Regional Children's Center. The model was developed based on an identified need to enhance collaborations between parents, teachers, and clinicians in helping school-age children with various forms of mental health or learning disabilities. The model is a method of integrated neuropsychological assessment, consultation, and intervention designed to improve parenting education and treatment effectiveness (Casey, Strang, Roach, & Innard, 1997; Strang, 1987). One part of this clinical model, the Neuropsychology School Conference (NSC), has been empirically tested and has received some preliminary empirical support (Casey et al., 1997). The utility of NCC lies in two main premises: the necessity for a child's parents, teachers, and clinicians to share a common understanding and realistic expectations of the child, and second, that remedial goals, intervention strategies, and environmental accommodations must be shared, coordinated, and implemented by these adults in the child's everyday environment (Casey et al., 1997).

The NCC model has developed over 20 years and reflects experiences in clinical practice from John Strang and colleagues. The feedback model involves three main phases: (1) listening to information provided by parents/guardians/loved ones about the child/patient in an initial neuropsychology interview session; (2) the second (post-testing) session involves connecting the neuropsychological assessment findings and implications to the information and perceptions provided by parents; (3) a similar exchange develops between parents and the child's teachers in the NSC. The advantage of this method is that parents enter the conference being more informed and educated about their child's condition and feel better equipped to dialogue with school officials about the child's capabilities and needs.

Experience with the model suggests that all team members, especially the child's parents, undergo a progressive building of understanding about the child's special strengths and needs throughout the implementation of the model. Furthermore, experience suggests that when all team members actively participate in the discussion and intervention plan generated at the NSC, a better and shared understanding of the child takes place. Anecdotal observations suggest that the child's day-to-day experiences have improved substantially, which can lead to dramatic improvements in the child's outlook.

Chapter 3
A Collaborative Therapeutic Neuropsychological Assessment Model

The Collaborative Therapeutic Neuropsychological Assessment (CTNA) model represents a hybrid clinical intervention that draws from the NAFI of Gorske and the CNA of Smith. Given their similar goals of increasing the clinical impact of neuropsychological assessment on patient well-being, feelings of responsibility and control, and life narrative, it seemed logical to combine the two into one comprehensive assessment intervention. Specifically, CTNA borrows its initial interview and general clinical approach from Smith's CNA, but the feedback and report are derived from Gorske's NAFI. The resultant product is both *collaborative* (in that the patient and the therapist work together to understand a particular set of life problems) and *therapeutic*, given that the ultimate goal is to reduce patient suffering or to help bring about a transformative experience.

Throughout this chapter, we generally refer to experiences, expectations, needs, and wishes of the patient. However, we acknowledge that in many neuropsychological cases, the patient may not be the *consumer* of the CTNA approach. When patients have experienced significant cognitive decline or injury, when the patient is a child, or when the patient is psychiatrically compromised, it is the patient's family who will be most directly involved. This does not mean that the CTNA approach is inappropriate or ineffectual, however. In all cases involving families, a collaborative approach that brings about a change in the way that a family views, understands, or treats a loved one can be extremely powerful and life changing. We will make such examples explicit in the following sections, but when we simply refer to *patients*, we have done so primarily for the sake of simplicity, not because we only think that patients are the only consumers of this intervention.

Last, there are some situations and settings in which the complete CTNA approach may not be appropriate or possible. In inpatient settings or in a consultation model in which testing is circumscribed and rapid or in which patients may be suffering from severe dementia, medical problems, or psychiatric involvement, the full model of CTNA, as we describe it, may not be practical. Furthermore, we know of some clinical settings where neuropsychologists are prohibited from providing test feedback directly to patients. However, a general collaborative approach with the patient is still relevant and important.

T.T. Gorske, S.R. Smith, *Collaborative Therapeutic Neuropsychological Assessment*, 39
DOI: 10.1007/978-0-387-75426-0_3, © Springer Science+Business Media, LLC 2009

Furthermore, given the importance of feedback in clinical practice (Allen et al., 1986; Gass & Brown, 1992; Lewak & Hogan, 2003), clinical neuropsychologists should look for ways that they can increase their impact and make their services relevant to patients they serve (Ruff, 2003).

Basic Assumptions of CTNA

This section will provide a set of basic assumptions that guide CTNA.

Assumption 1: The patient/caregiver/referral source has noticed a change in the patient's cognitive and/or behavioral functioning and would like a professional to tell if there is a true change, to what degree, how severe, its potential causes, and outlook for the future. CTNA operates under the assumption that patients or supportive others are looking for information that can explain changes they are experiencing in their daily lives. And even if there has not been a change in the patient's behavior, there might now be a mismatch between a patient's functioning and the demands of their environment (e.g., a child begins to show signs of a learning disability in school). Historically, neuropsychological information was hidden from patients and caregivers, and it was often left to the referring provider to interpret the results and use them for the benefit of the patient. However, this places the patient and supportive others in a passive situation where they have little to no input into how the information is used and therefore do not have a voice in their care. CTNA follows patient-centered methods of care, where patients and supportive others are active collaborators and empowered to be involved in the testing and use of results. CTNA works to meet this need for knowledge and empowerment through an open sharing of neuropsychological test results.

Assumption 2: The patient/family members are distressed because of the change in the patient's cognitive/behavioral functioning. Part of the reason they are coming in for the evaluation is to receive help, direction, and guidance in order to feel less distressed. Changes in cognitive functioning and the confusion created by the change can lead to emotional distress and fear in patients. Essentially, it is the fear of the unknown. Not knowing what's "going on inside your own head" can be frightening, because patients often catastrophize by thinking more is wrong with them than there really is. For example, patients who are depressed and experience information processing slowing, attention, working memory, and general memory difficulties, may fear that they have a tumor, Alzheimer's disease, or some other horrible illness. CTNA seeks to alleviate patient distress by providing concrete information in a way that is understandable. The provision of knowledge can provide guidance and direction and begin alleviating fears of the unknown while clarifying misconceptions that feed these fears.

Assumption 3: So that they might feel better about themselves, patients would like to know of potential ameliorative strategies so that they are able to perform better in school, work, and social spheres. Patients who are confused, scared, and distressed want to feel better. In general, patients who have knowledge, guidance, and direction begin to feel less distressed and more in control of their lives. One of the goals of CTNA is to provide recommendations for treatment or rehabilitation that are individualized. Patients are more likely to follow through with recommendations if they have been active collaborators in the decision-making process and have a voice in what type of treatment they feel would be most helpful. In CTNA, recommendations are individualized, and one of the first questions asked is "How would you like to use this information?" When standard, prescribed rehabilitation recommendations are given (e.g., a cholinesterase inhibitor for an elderly patient with mild cognitive impairment; cognitive therapy for a patient who is depressed, academic tutoring for a child with dyslexia, or cognitive rehabilitation for a TBI patient), patients are more likely to consider such recommendations if they have been actively involved in the decision-making process and they feel the recommendations have been individualized to fit their needs.

Assumption 4: *Although patients seek guidance and direction from the psychologist, they also want to be respected and to be empowered as active and autonomous participants in treatment and decision-making processes.* This assumption best describes the core foundation as to why CTNA is important. Adherence to treatment regimens is a problematic issue in health care. Despite advances in scientific, and more specifically neuropsychological, knowledge, patients often do not follow through with recommendations from health-care professionals. One reason is that patients do not believe they have been empowered to be active participants in their own health-care decisions. A basic philosophy of CTNA is that an informed, educated, and empowered patient will be actively involved in their health care and are more likely to trust and respect professional recommendations. Consequently, they may be more likely to adhere to suggested treatment regimens.

Assumption 5: *Neuropsychological tests provide objective, concrete information about patients' cognitive and behavioral functioning that applies to their daily life and problems they may be experiencing.* There is evidence from both research and experience that neuropsychological tests are valid measures of individuals' functional abilities (Lezak, Howieson, & Loring, 2004; Meyer et al., 2001). Neuropsychological tests measure skills most people use on a daily basis, but take them for granted. Often, patients will report feeling disorganized, unable to focus and pay attention, unable to remember things, or having trouble making decisions. Difficulties with these cognitive skills have a reciprocal relationship between patients' moods and consequent life stressors.

For example, consider a patient who is depressed because she believes that she is worthless. Her depression leads to difficulties with focusing and concentrating, which affect her work performance. Her impaired work performance reinforces her belief that she is worthless, which further exacerbates her depression and ability to focus. Her poor concentration worsens to the point where she believes she is flawed and defective and may have brain damage. The negative beliefs and depression are now so deep that she only feels relief from drinking alcohol and being drunk.

In this case, the patient could benefit from hearing that she is not flawed, defective, or brain damaged but that her attention and focusing problems are likely due to depression, and some antidepressants and psychotherapy may begin to help her feel better by challenging her negative beliefs. This example illustrates the generalizability of neuropsychological tests to everyday life and the reciprocal nature of cognitive and emotional problems.

Assumption 6: Feedback to patients from neuropsychological tests can help answer questions regarding changes in cognitive and behavioral functioning, provide hypotheses as to the causes of these changes, and give direction for treatment planning or rehabilitation. This assumption speaks of the benefit of feedback, specifically neuropsychological feedback, in enhancing patient care. The exact mechanisms that make feedback effective are not well understood. Experience and research suggest that feedback may be effective because the information provided can change patient's attitudes and beliefs about their health and may motivate them to make changes that are perceived as necessary. Furthermore, feedback allows patients to change their cognitive narratives in a way that helps them have a more complex understanding of their strengths and weaknesses, the origins or their deficits, and their ability to care for themselves and plan for the future. In addition, the comparison to social norms may facilitate motivation to make changes (DiClemente, Marinilli, Singh, & Bellino, 2001). However, the provision of information is not sufficient in and of itself, which leads to the final assumption.

Assumption 7: Feedback presented in a patient-centered manner can elicit the patient as an active collaborator, empower them in the treatment and decision-making process, and lower resistance to hearing difficult or discrepant information. This will motivate them to work closely with professionals to alleviate their problems and distress. Information and feedback that are provided in the context of a supportive and helping relationship that respects patient perceptions and autonomy are more likely to be heard and used than feedback that is given in an authoritative "top-down" manner, where a patient is told what to do and offered a prescriptive treatment plan without consideration for their individual needs. CTNA individualizes neuropsychological information by applying the information to patients' lives and functioning while enlisting them as active decision-makers in the treatment-planning process. CTNA empowers patients by giving them valuable knowledge about themselves, their behavior, and their functioning. With CTNA, patients are empowered to use the knowledge for their benefit and they decide, with help and guidance from professionals, how they would like to use the information they learn.

A key component is the patient-centered interpersonal nature of the clinician. Clinicians provide feedback in a manner that conveys respect and empathy for the patient. The patient is seen as the expert on themselves, while the clinician has knowledge and expertise that may help explain aspects of the patient's cognitive and behavioral functioning. The clinician freely imparts this information to the patients and gives the message that the patient is empowered and ultimately responsible for how they use this information. Thus, the patient and clinician contribute their individual knowledge in a collaborative effort to help the patient understand themselves and make any important changes that might be necessary. This type of collaborative, patient-centered approach has shown to lower patient's resistance to hearing information that might otherwise be difficult for them to take in (Finn, 2007). Ultimately, patients feel empowered to accept or reject the information. However, experience suggests that when patients are empowered and initiated as collaborators, they are more likely to accept information.

Chapter 4
The Initial Interview: Collaborative Information Gathering

In this chapter we provide a brief overview of the initial interviewing process and discuss the importance of gathering relevant information in a collaborative manner. This is not meant to be a chapter on interviewing techniques, as there are many definitive books that adequately describe such methods (e.g., Adams, Parson, Culbertson, & Nixon, 1996; Green, 2000; Groth-Marnat, 2003). This chapter is meant to provide some principles of conducting an interview in a collaborative manner that enlist the patient as an active participant in the interviewing process. The perspective is that the patient, and/or their family, are the best source of information that will guide the assessment and eventual feedback.

Before progressing further, it is important to define what is meant by "the patient and/or their family are the best sources of information." On the surface, this might sound like an overreliance on patient/family self-report when this may not be the best source of accurate information about many patients' clinical presentation. This may be true in many cases; however, to understand the importance of the patient/family as the best source of information, it is important to differentiate between objective and subjective (phenomenological) information and the value of each.

Objective information simply refers to essential clinical data that aids in the formulation of a diagnosis. This includes, but is not limited to, facts of the case, historical information related to the current clinical presentation, patient behavioral responses, collateral information from significant others or referral sources, medical records, results from objective tests, and many others. Most astute clinicians are competent in gathering this information and using it to aid in diagnostic formulations and deciding the best test protocol to administer. This information is what typically goes into the report and is given back to referral sources and sometimes to patients. It is consistent with the "Information Gathering" model of assessment and could be considered the "gold standard" for data gathering and history taking. The advantage of gathering objective information is that it allows for a comprehensive analysis of all the factors that may contribute to a neuropsychological phenomenon. In addition, it is a simply good and ethical psychological interviewing. Most patients expect this type of experience from health professionals, so they are not surprised when they experience

T.T. Gorske, S.R. Smith, *Collaborative Therapeutic Neuropsychological Assessment*,
DOI: 10.1007/978-0-387-75426-0_4, © Springer Science+Business Media, LLC 2009

such a session. The disadvantage of objective information gathering is that it often misses the individual experience of the person as a potential source of valuable information. In addition, patients often leave such an interview feeling dissected, as if they were a lab animal being studied, not a person being heard. It is this latter case, a person who is understood, seen, and heard, that describes a more subjective, collaborative, information gathering.

Collaborative interviewing views the patient's subjective experience of a problem or complaint as equally important as the facts of the case. Examples of a patients' subjective experience includes their feelings about a problem, their perception of what the problem means, their hopes and dreams for how the problem will be solved or coped with, and the ways they hope professionals and significant others can help them resolve or cope with the problem. The advantage of this approach is that patients often have the experience of being understood and valued. Patients experience their thoughts and opinions as important, and they often want to share more of themselves.

The result of this collaborative style can be that the patient feels comfortable providing more information that is clinically useful, and it helps the clinician view the patient holistically rather than reducing them to a list of traits, diagnoses, and constructs. This can also go a long way in reducing patient's resistance to the testing experience. Consider the following example with an elderly patient referred for testing to provide further evidence for a suspected diagnosis of dementia. The patient was angry and suspicious about the testing and continually voiced her displeasure at the examiner for "making her do things".

Examiner: Ok Margaret, what I'd like to talk about is how you see yourself doing with things like shopping. Are you doing your own shopping and do you notice any changes in how that goes?

Patient: Oh, I do fine. I don't see why I have to answer that. Why are you making me answer these things?

Examiner: It seems insulting to you?

Patient: Yes it does! I've never been through something like this in my life. Why do I have to go through this?

Examiner: It seems pointless to you that people are making you do this.

Patient: Yes, I don't know why all this is happening. I raised my children all my life and now I'm being treated like some sort of invalid!

Examiner: They don't trust you can take care of yourself.

Patient: I took care of *them* all my life. Do you know I was one of the few girls with a diploma on my block? My children knew their mother had it upstairs. So did the others where we lived. All those years I worked I had to use my smarts. I even worked for the first few years after my firstborn. My husband didn't want me to but I said to hell with him.

Examiner: So it's a mystery why they won't let you do the things you used to do?

Patient: Yeah, they don't trust me now.

Examiner: Did something happen?
Patient: Oh if it did, I'm sure my daughter would tell you. She seems to
                 have a handle on things
Examiner: She's a smart cookie, just like her mother.
Patient: Yeah (laughs).
Examiner: Is she doing the shopping for you now?
Patient: Yes. She doesn't trust me anymore.

Here, instead of repeatedly barraging the patient with questions, the examiner takes time to assess the patient's experience of what is happening in her life. In doing so, a clinical description of the patient becomes more apparent, but more than that, the patient begins to view the examiner as an ally rather than another person "doing things to her" and becomes more amenable to sharing information she is able to recall. The result of this interview was that through continually validating the patient's experience, the examiner facilitated her motivation to complete the tests, which became a testament to her energy and motivation to follow through with tasks when encouraged. Although this particular patient was eventually diagnosed as suffering from dementia, the resources and strengths she displayed through a validating environment served to develop treatment plans for helping her family and caregivers capitalize on her strengths as a way to cope with her deficits.

This leads to another reason that it is important to evaluate patients' emotional experience of their problem. Imagine two patients who have recently suffered from traumatic brain injuries. One patient, Mike, speaks mournfully about the loss of function that he has experienced, his loss of work, and strained relationships with his family and friends. Another patient, David, has experienced the same setbacks and changes as Mike. However, during the interview he discusses how he is grateful to be alive and, although saddened by his problems, seems to have energy to contribute to all aspects of his rehabilitation. Even if we assume that both of these patients have experienced the same losses, we can see that David has a much better prognosis. We can expect that he will be an active and aggressive participant in his rehabilitation and that the treatment team will rally in his support.

A collaborative interviewing style can allow us to see how our patients' subjective reality will shape and interact with their rehabilitation, treatment, or remediation. Their experience of their problems also shapes and gives expression to their symptoms. We know that people who are depressed and anxious will often have more somatic complaints than people who do not. In the same manner, our patients' personality styles, affect, interpersonal expectations, and coping systems will shape the way that their neuropsychological symptoms are expressed and understood. An evaluation of patients' emotional resilience will allow clinicians to add a depth of understanding to the test results that cannot be simply communicated through scores and historical facts alone.

Conducting the Initial Interview

There are three main components of the initial interview in a collaborative approach: (1) understanding the problem, when it occurs and for how long; (2) understanding the patient's emotional experience of the problem; and (3) understanding the patient's wishes for the assessment, results, and outcomes.

Understanding the Problem

Generally speaking, this is a gathering of background information. The important part is to understand this information from the patient's and the family's perspectives. Beyond simply evaluating the basic presence of symptoms and a laundry list of problems, the goal of this portion of the interview is to understand the symptoms in context of the patient's day-to-day life and that of their family and loved ones. For example, the loss of some fine motor control might be difficult for an attorney, but it would be devastating for a concert pianist. Once this portion of the interview is complete, you will have not only a detailed clinical history but also the history from the patient's perspective, in their own words.

One method for doing this is to obtain clinical information with a questioning style that balances close-ended, fact-finding questions with more open-ended elaborative questions. Consider the following examples:

Close-ended dialogue

Examiner: Do you have any medical problems?
Patient: No
Examiner: Have you had any past medical problems?
Patient: Like what?
Examiner: Like head injuries, periods of unconsciousness, seizures, comas, problematic surgeries, major health problems that affected your ability to function?
Patient: Not that I can recall.

Open-Ended dialogue

Examiner: Tell me about your medical history.
Patient: Like what?
Examiner: Well, it could be anything that sticks out for you. For example, tell me about any times you experienced a head injury.
Patient: Does a car accident count?
Examiner: It could, sure. Can you tell me more about that?

Patient: Well, I was a passenger while my buddy and I were driving around while I was in college. We got rear-ended by another car and my head hit the windshield pretty good.
Examiner: Wow! What happened?
Patient: Well, I think I might have been out for a while because the next thing I remember is being in the hospital.
Examiner: What do you recall the doctors saying about your condition?
Patient: Something about a concussion. Oh . . . I remember they said something about a closed head injury and I got CP or CV scan or something like that.
Examiner: It sounds really scary. What was all that like for you?
Patient: I was pretty freaked. I was really out of it partly because I think they might have had me on something. I remember not being right for about one or two weeks after that.

The main advantages of an open-ended approach are that it requires the patient to elaborate on what they are saying and provides more information than might be gathered with close-ended questions. In addition, by asking the patient their reactions to situations, you can gauge the contribution of the patient's emotional experience to the situation at hand.

Understanding the effect of the problem on family members is also important. This is particularly true when working with children and adolescents. The basic question an examiner wants to know is what are the real-world consequences of the problem? An example of an interview dialogue might be as follows:

Examiner: So you say it takes four hours for Brian to complete his homework each night. What effect does this have on everyone else in the family?
Parents: Well, you can imagine that it's a real nightmare each night.
Examiner: How so?
Parent: Well, it certainly gets in the way of other activities that are important to the family. Before all of this started, we used to have dinner and relax as a family. Now my wife and I spend all of our time pushing Brian to do his work. We're always nagging him and riding him. His sister Julie feels completely ignored and she'll get so mad that she'll throw temper tantrums – and that certainly doesn't help calm everyone down.
Examiner: How are you all dealing with this?
Parent: It's really taking a toll on our marriage and the kids see us fight a lot these days.

You can see from this example that Brian's cognitive issue (a possible learning disability) affects not only his ability to function in school but also the functioning of his entire family. Furthermore, as his family becomes more and more stressed, it is likely to further disrupt his ability to perform at his best.

All problems exist in a context, and that context will exert its own pressure on the situation.

Understanding the Emotional Experience of the Problem

In a collaborative interview process, it is important to keep a focus on the emotional experience of the problem.; that is, what is the effect of the problem on the patient's subjective experience of themselves, their lives and relationships, and their future? This is important because it allows us to gain an understanding of how the patient's subjective experience may be affecting the results of the testing and what that might mean for treatment and rehabilitation planning. Consider the following example:

Mr. J, a man, in his early 30s, who recently underwent brain surgery to remove a tumor, was undergoing neuropsychological testing to determine if the surgery had affected his cognition. The surgery was successful, and there were no reports of subjective cognitive complaints. In performing the Rey–Osterrieth Complex Figure, the patient displayed a high degree of anxiety, perseverated over many of the design details, and showed difficulty in planning and organizing the details into a coherent whole. His immediate and delayed recalls of the design were impaired. Specifically, he could not remember many of the details, although his basic memory for the gestalt of the design was relatively intact. An initial impression was that his pattern of deficits was consistent with the site of the tumor. However, in further discussing the patient's performance, he stated that the test tapped into his perfectionist tendencies, which were present prior to the development of the tumor. He was highly anxious about being able to reconstruct the drawing correctly, and his performance anxiety did not allow him to process the information efficiently. As a result, he was overly focused on minute details and did not remember how the design was constructed.

This example illustrates the importance of considering a patient's subjective experience of the problem. Furthermore, it is imperative to evaluate how they cope with any new problems or ongoing cognitive issues. As was discussed above, patients' coping styles will shape how their problems are expressed and will dictate their prognosis. Examples of questions to ask include the following:

- How are you coping with all of these changes?
- Tell me more about how you see your future.
- What's it like to see other students doing their work so easily when it's so hard for you?
- What do you look forward to?

After learning the basic background information of the problem, when it occurs, and how it affects the lives of your patient and/or their family, you should be able to form an interpretation of the patient's Central Cognitive-Emotional Complaint (CCEC).

The Central Cognitive-Emotional Complaint

The CCEC is a concept new to the CTNA approach. It is based on Luborsky's (1984) model of the therapeutic Core Conflictual Relationship Theme. Luborsky's work pioneered manualized short-term dynamic psychotherapy. His CCRT treatment is an often used and researched method of understanding maladaptive object relations and providing succinct interpretations of interpersonal problems.

We have borrowed Luborsky's model and adapted it to be appropriate for a neuropsychological assessment interview. The goal is to empathetically reflect an understanding of the patient's experience in a neuropsychological context. The CCEC is a succinct way of summarizing the patient's problem and how it makes the patient or the patient's family feel. It allows the clinician to quickly summarize (and check) their understanding of the problem and its real-life consequences. There are three components to the CCEC:

1. The patients' wish or desire for themselves and/or their lives (W);
2. A behavioral or cognitive reaction (this is merely a statement of the patient's experienced difficulty: CR);
3. An emotional response to that difficulty (ER).

Some examples of the CCEC might be as follows:

Examiner: From what we've discussed here today, it seems that you want Brian to have a better experience of school (W), but that he really struggles with paying attention in the classroom and at home during homework (CR). It sounds like that really makes him down on himself and even takes a toll on the family (ER). Does that sound about right?

Examiner: From what we discussed here today, it seems like you really want to succeed in school (W), but that no matter how hard you try, you're not really able to perform as quickly as the other kids (CR), and that really frustrates you (ER).

Examiner: Let me see if I understand everything so far. Since the injury, you've had a hard time with so many things that used to come so easily (CR). Because you want so badly to feel like yourself again (W), you find yourself getting upset and taking it out on your wife (ER).

Examiner: It sounds like you really want the best for your Mom (W). But these things you've noticed recently – the forgetfulness, the confusion, and the falls (CR) – really have you concerned about her future and her ability to care for herself (ER). I often meet with families who are facing the same types of questions and I'm glad to see that you're so supportive and invested. Hopefully, the results of testing will be another piece in the puzzle so that we can figure out what's going on.

There are a number of advantages to developing the CCEC in this way. First, it helps the patient or the patient's family feel as though their problems and perceptions are understood. This serves to enhance rapport building and patient self-disclosure. Second, the evaluator begins to understand the multiple factors that influence the nature of a problem. The problem is understood not only from a discrete brain–behavior relationship perspective but also from a contextual perspective. There are many factors that influence cognitive processes. The advantage of developing the CCEC is that you are able to understand a range of factors that may be potentially influencing a problem, and these factors will go into your analysis, conclusions, and treatment recommendations.

Furthermore, the CCEC allows the patient or family to disagree with your initial formulation. We might often be too quick to put patients into discrete boxes of "Alzheimer's patient," "learning disabled," or "brain injured." In addition to merely dehumanizing patients, this type of shorthand might truly miss the real of the most pressing issue facing the family. We must always be open to being "set straight" by a patient or family who feels misunderstood or misread. It's important that we don't let busy schedules, time constraints, or referring provider diagnoses cloud our judgment of a clinical situation.

The CCEC acts as a natural segue into the third domain of the initial interview. Now that the nature of the cognitive-emotional concerns has been identified, a discussion about how the assessment can serve to resolve this issue can commence.

Understanding the Patient's Wishes for the Assessment, Results, and Outcomes

The goal of this process is to understand what the patient really wants and expects from the assessment so as to clarify expectations. As part of this process, it may be helpful to ask the patient to develop up to three questions they hope can be answered by the evaluation. This can be done at the end of the initial interview and revisited prior to the feedback session. It can often happen that a patient or patient's family has questions and expectations of the assessment that are unrealistic. As psychologists, we are often asked what type of medications might be appropriate, how much more rehabilitation might be needed, whether the condition is genetic, or if the condition might be caused by another medical issue. Consider the following example:

Patient's Parent: I'm really hoping that you can tell me about what types of medication would best help Rachael.

Examiner:	That's a great question, but one that I will not be able to answer for you. Testing will help us better understand what's going on with Rachael and where her strengths and weaknesses are, but questions about medi-cation should be answered by a physician, preferably a psychiatrist. If, at the end of this evaluation, you're still interested in learning about pharmacological treatment, we'll be happy to pro-vide you with some referrals. For now, let's talk a little bit more about your concerns about Rachael and your reasons for feeling that she may need medication. Are there other questions that you have about Rachael's performance at school or her behavior at home that we may be able to help you with through this assessment?

Although we *may* have opinions about these issues such as medication, it is important to let the patient know when their questions will not be answered by neuropsychological testing. Helping them reframe their questions to be more consistent with the goals and products of assessment will reduce feelings of disappointment and frustration prior to the evaluation.

An important part of the initial interview conclusion is to socialize the patient regarding the process of neuropsychological assessment. Psychotherapy research indicates that socializing patients to the process and roles of psychotherapy reduces dropout and improves alliance (Book, 1998; Heitler, 1973; Luborsky, 1984; Reis & Brown, 1999). Given that the CNA is an approach to improve a feeling of collaboration, it is important to socialize the patient and/or patient's family to the process of neuropsychological assessment. Although it is not necessary to describe, in detail, each and every procedure, it is important to let patients know how long testing will last as well as the types of tasks they'll be expected to perform. A discussion to normalize any potential feelings of failure and frustration will also help the patient feel better prepared and fully engaged in the process. An example of a statement used to socialize patients may be as follows:

"Let me take a few minutes to tell you what to expect from today. I'm going to ask you a number of things in order to try to answer your questions. We begin with an evaluation of your global cognitive functioning. Put another way, how are you doing in the broadest sense? Then, because you have concerns about [a particular cognitive issue] we're going to do lots of tests that will require you to pay attention to things, solve problems, organize, etc. Last, we're going to take some time to see how you are doing psychologically. This is so we can see if there's a connection between how you think and feel. Do you have any questions so far? Most people find the tests interesting and sometimes even enjoyable, others find them boring, stressful, or taxing. Some things will be very easy, others may be harder than you expect. Also there may be times you don't think you're doing as well as you should be. It's normal to feel that way. An important thing is that I won't be able to tell you how you're doing during the evaluation, but I will always need you to try your best. Any questions about that? Now it's going to be a long day, but we'll take lots of breaks. If you need to rest or stop, please let me know. Once we're through, I will take all the tests and score them. Your score will be compared to scores from thousands of other people across the country. That way, we can tell if your score falls in the average range. Afterwards I will write two reports. One report is a "technical report" that is read by other professionals. The other is more patient-friendly that will explain the results in a meaningful way for you. You'll get both of those reports when we meet for the feedback session in about a month. At that time, we'll discuss the results and think about ways to use them to make any changes and develop a treatment plan. Do you have any questions about that or anything else I've mentioned?"

Another method is to give patients a one-page copy of a form briefly describing neuropsychological assessment in layman's terms, such as the form generated from the federally funded study evaluating the effects of neuropsychological assessment feedback on patient outcomes (NAFI, described in previous chapters. See form in Appendix A).

Summary and Moving to the Assessment

The initial interview is the place to "set the stage" for a collaborative neuropsychological assessment. In addition to gathering important clinical information, the examiner gains an understanding of the patient's subjective experience of the problem that brings them in for a neuropsychological assessment. This is important for a number of reasons. First, it helps establish rapport and lowers patient resistance and suspiciousness about the assessment process. This can facilitate self-disclosure, comfort with the examiner, and create a general feeling of mutual understanding, respect, and collaboration where the examiner and patient can feel as if they are working together to understand the nature of the problem. Second, the patient can begin to feel like an active participant in the process as opposed to being a passive recipient. Constance Fisher describes this as the patient being a co-facilitator and co-interpreter of the assessment process. Such an approach encourages patient empowerment where patients become active initiators of their own health care. Patient-centered models of medicine have shown that such an approach leads patients to be better health-care consumers who take active steps in their own health-care decisions and can potentially lead to more health-conducive behaviors. This is the outcome desired for collaborative neuropsychological assessment, where patients feel empowered to be active participants in the process and become motivated to take steps to improve their own outcomes. Finally, this approach satisfies an ethical obligation of psychologists to fully inform patients about the nature and results of psychological test procedures (Pope, 1992; APA, 2002).

Many neuropsychologists have offered stories where, despite their best efforts, patients leave an assessment and feedback process feeling unsatisfied and "talked down to." In rare cases this has led to ethical complaints against psychologists who appeared to be acting in a patient's best interest. A collaborative approach attempts to ensure active patient involvement throughout the entire process and may decrease the likelihood that a patient feels disempowered and lodges a complaint.

From this point, the neuropsychological assessment process proceeds in the standard manner, with standardized procedures using whatever battery is deemed appropriate. Experience from clinical practice and formal research suggests that when patients are initiated to the process through the collaborative interview method, they are more motivated to initiate and complete the process. Often, many patients who undergo neuropsychological assessments continue to remain "in the dark" in regard to the purpose of the assessment and what information will be gained to improve the quality of their lives. Experience suggests that patients who are part of a collaborative interview, approach the assessment with a sense of inquisitiveness and an understanding that the assessment is designed to provide answers to difficult questions. They have the sense that they are working together with their clinician to discover previously unknown things about themselves. In addition, the patient feels empowered to be a part of the process and acts as a co-initiator versus a passive recipient.

Chapter 5
The CTNA Feedback Session

This chapter will illustrate the process and structure of a CTNA feedback session. The first section will discuss the overarching conceptual framework on which a feedback session is based. The subsequent sections will describe the methods for conducting a CTNA feedback session.

CTNA Feedback Conceptual Basis

In order to conduct a CTNA feedback session, a clinician must understand the CTNA conceptual basis. As reviewed in the background literature, CTNA is based on three primary approaches. The first is therapeutic/individual models of psychological assessment, primarily from the work of Dr. Constance Fischer and Dr. Stephen Finn. Second are recommendations from authors on the provision of neuropsychological test feedback. Third, the principles of Motivational Interviewing (MI) as reflected in the personalized feedback report and the format for providing information, which is termed "Elicit–Provide–Elicit."

Therapeutic/Individualized Models of Psychological Assessment

The primary components of these models that form the basis for CTNA are that psychological assessment and feedback are (1) a collaboration between tester and examinee, (2) open and flexible with a mutual sharing of information, (3) consider patient opinions about the nature of testing results, (4) view testing results in the context of the patient's life, and (5) see the test results as a "snapshot" of the patient's life and general functioning, and that test results are tools that are used to help understand a patient holistically.

T.T. Gorske, S.R. Smith, *Collaborative Therapeutic Neuropsychological Assessment,*   57
DOI: 10.1007/978-0-387-75426-0_5, © Springer Science+Business Media, LLC 2009

Neuropsychological Test Feedback Recommendations

The next component of the model includes recommendations from authors for giving neuropsychological test feedback that is applicable, useful, and relevant to patients (Armengol et al., 2001; Gass & Brown, 1992; Pope, 1992). These include the following principles: (1) the purpose of neuropsychological testing and the results should be reviewed in plain, simple language understandable to the patient, (2) test results are examples of functioning and behavior that may contribute to understanding other life areas, (3) results are termed as strengths or weaknesses compared to available standard norms, and (4) test results can help develop useful and applicable treatment plans that consider the domains of functioning assessed.

Motivational Interviewing Principles (Miller and Rollnick, 2002)

The final component includes specific methods from MI. The first is the framework for providing feedback termed "Elicit–Provide–Elicit". Second, MI describes specific verbal skills for interacting with patients in a patient-centered and directive manner, termed OARS (*open-ended questions, affirmations, reflections, and summarizations*). Third, MI provides specific recommendations for dealing with resistance and includes various directive and nondirective strategies all designed to "roll with resistance." We will elaborate on these concepts in greater depth.

MI is a patient-centered and directive form of counseling designed to enhance patient's internal motivation to make changes in problematic behaviors. Originally developed to treat patients with alcoholism, MI represented a paradigm shift from the traditional "confrontation of denial of approach." In this approach, patients with alcoholism are assumed to be in denial about the effects of alcoholism on their lives. Therefore, a counselor's job is to "break the denial" through highly challenging and sometimes harsh methods of making patients see the reality of their situation. MI philosophy states that this is unnecessary to enact the change process and that the goal is to lower patient resistance through nondirective strategies, and it identifies patient's ambivalence about making changes. Once the ambivalence, or the conflict, about making change is identified, the counselor uses any number of techniques to help the patient resolve the ambivalence and move toward making important and necessary changes. One method used in MI is the provision of objective feedback from various psychosocial measures. MI authors have developed an explicit and concrete conceptual framework for providing feedback in a patient-centered manner. These principles are highly consistent with previous authors' ideas of ways to use psychological test feedback. This section will provide a brief overview of MI principles including methods for providing objective feedback. This will include a brief literature review of the evidence of efficacy for the provision of feedback in an MI style. Most of the information will be based on the groundbreaking work of Dr. William Miller and Dr. Stephen Rollnick (Miller & Rollnick, 1991, 2002).

MI is a brief intervention designed to enhance treatment adherence in patients with various health or mental health problems. MI was developed to enhance treatment adherence in patients with alcoholism but over the last 15 years has shown to be effective in enhancing patients' motivation to change drug use, health behaviors such as following diabetic regimens, improving medication compliance, and others (Miller & Rollnick, 1991, 2002; Hettema, Steele, & Miller, 2005; Resnicow et al., 2002).

MI is more a method of dialogue than a theory, and the mechanisms of action are not well understood; however, it is based on well-established theoretical principles (Hettema et al., 2005). MI is heavily based on Carl Rogers' necessary and sufficient conditions for establishing a therapeutic relationship; empathy, congruence, and respect (Rogers, 1951). Empathy and reflective listening are the heart of MI, where the goal is to understand the patient's point of view regarding a problematic behavior they are trying to change. Empathy and respect by the clinician are hypothesized to lower a patient's resistance to making changes and allows for the exploration of ambivalence (Miller & Rollnick, 1991, 2002; Moyers & Rollnick, 2002). MI principles suggest that most patients are ambivalent about making changes in their behavior, as opposed to being completely resistant or completely ready to make changes. Exploring and resolving ambivalence is a key goal in MI. The exploration and resolving of ambivalence has roots in Festinger's Cognitive Dissonance Theory and Bem's Self-Perception Theory (Bem, 1967; Festinger, 1957). One of the MI principles is to develop a discrepancy between a patient's behavior and their personal goals or values. The patient will then become uncomfortable and begin to take steps toward resolving the discrepancy, which is hypothesized to move in the direction of growth and change. Finally, MI is associated with the "stages of change" conceptual framework, which posits that patients change problematic behavior through a sequence of stages. These stages are precontemplation (change is not considered), contemplation (change is considered), preparation (a commitment to change is made), action (change is enacted), maintenance, and relapse prevention where ongoing change is fostered (Miller & Rollnick, 1991, 2002; Prochaska, DiClemente, & Norcross, 1992).

MI's conceptual basis can be summarized in four principles: (1) a counselor expresses *empathy* for a patient, which creates an atmosphere of safety and promotes self-focus and disclosure; (2) a counselor *develops discrepancy* between the patient's behavior and important goals or values; (3) a counselor avoids argumentation and *rolls with resistance* versus imposing change strategies; and (4) a counselor supports a patient's *self-efficacy* to resolve problems (Miller & Rollnick, 1991, 2002). MI is a humanistic/phenomenological intervention because the clinician works to enter the patient's individual world before making any attempts to enact change strategies.

MI shares methods identified as effective in other brief therapies. These methods are captured in the acronym FRAMES. Patient's receive personalized *F*eedback from objective measures in order to gain insight and awareness; clinicians emphasize a patient's personal *R*esponsibility in making changes in their lives; clinicians may offer *A*dvice on ways patients can begin to make changes; advice may be given as a *M*enu of alternatives for making behavioral changes; a clinician is always *E*mpathizing with a patient's perspective; and finally, clinicians seek to enhance a patients *S*elf-efficacy in their ability to make changes(Miller & Rollnick, 1991/2002).

The Feedback Process in MI

The provision of objective feedback is one method used in MI to enhance problem recognition. The most common use of feedback is the personalized feedback report. The feedback report gives patients information about their severity of substance use, general functional abilities, DSM-IV diagnoses, frequency of drinking and other drug use compared to national norms, and occasionally, the results from very brief neuropsychological tests (Miller et al., 1992). In MI, feedback is given in an objective, nonjudgmental manner that is designed to enhance the therapeutic dialogue. The conceptual framework for providing feedback, information, and advice is termed, "Elicit–Provide–Elicit." A clinician *elicits* a patient's commitment to engage in the feedback process and asks permission to provide the patient information that may be useful to them. Upon receiving the patient's agreement, the clinician *provides* information that is related to the patient's concerns and is designed to facilitate the change process. This information may include results from objective feedback reports and assessment results. After providing the information, the clinician *elicits* a patient's reaction to hearing the information. The clinician then responds to the patient's reactions with reflective listening, affirmations, summarizations of the patient's statements, and open-ended questions to encourage elaborations. If patients disagree with the results, become angry, or question the feedback validity, the clinician does not become defensive or try to justify the results. In MI, clinicians "role with resistance," which means they meet resistance with understanding, empathy and open-ended and evocative questions designed to clarify the nature of the resistance. The belief is that by lowering resistance through nondirective methods, patients become more open to exploration of ambivalence and begin to experience a discrepancy between their behavior and their goals and values. The clinician's goal is then to help patients work through and resolve ambivalence and move through the stages of change to enhance motivation to change a problematic behavior (Miller & Rollnick, 1991, 2002).

Evidence for the Effectiveness of Brief Feedback

There is evidence that brief feedback is effective in enhancing outcomes. A review of 13 studies examining the use of feedback as an alcohol intervention for college students concluded that feedback has modest support in the literature for changing drinking behavior (Walters & Neighbors, 2005). Feedback was hypothesized to be effective because college students learned how their behavior compared to similar norm groups. The most common feedback mechanism is the drinker's checkup, where patients are given objective feedback about their risk of developing alcohol-related problems (Hester, Squires, & Delaney, 2005; Miller, Sovereign, & Krege, 1988). Most studies using objective feedback delivered in the style of MI have shown good outcomes for reducing alcohol-related risk factors, improving treatment compliance, and making changes in health habits (Barrowclough et al., 2001; Bien, Miller, & Boroughs, 1993; Carroll, Libby, Sheehan, & Hyland, 2001; Daley, Salloum, Zuckoff, Kirisci, & Thase, 1998; Martino, Carroll, O'Malley, & Rounsaville, 2000; Miller, Benefield, & Tonigan, 1993; Stotts, Schmitz, Rhoades, & Grabowski, 2001; Swanson, Pantalon, & Cohen, 1999). A limitation of these studies is that it is difficult to discern whether the effect is from the feedback or from the MI style of delivery. A common practice is to adapt the personalized feedback report in order to meet the needs of the patient population being studied. Variables incorporated into feedback reports may include information about substance use frequencies, motivation, psychiatric symptoms, medical factors, and others (Martino et al., 2000; Miller et al., 1993; Stotts et al., 2001). In studies conducted in Addiction Medicine Services at Western Psychiatric Institute and Clinic, feedback forms were adapted for dual-disorder patients based on diagnostic symptoms; scores from a measure of functional behavior called the Addiction Severity Index; scores from the Drinker Inventory of Consequences (DRINC), which measures various psychosocial and interpersonal consequences from substance use; and comparisons of drinking frequencies to national norms. Occasionally, psychological measures of personality or cognitive functioning may be used, but these are not primary feedback tools in MI.

In summary, MI principles for the provision of patient-centered, objective feedback share many concepts with other author's previous ideas on ways to provide information from the results of psychological and neuropsychological tests. Miller and Rollnick have elucidated a process for providing patient-centered feedback with a clear and concrete method. The strength of this approach is that different types of information can be nested within the feedback method. A personalized feedback report can be modified to meet the needs of the examiner or the patient.

These three primary components comprise the conceptual basis for the CTNA feedback session. The most important notion is that the clinician and patient are working together to understand the patient's functioning from a holistic perspective. Rather than just relaying test scores and performance, the clinician's task is to help patients make sense of their difficulties by offering them a "snapshot" of their cognitive and behavioral functioning. Conversely, the patient's job is to help the clinician make sense of the test scores in the context of the patient's real world.

The Format of a CTNA Feedback Session

Step 1: Setting the Agenda and Introducing the Feedback Report

The first step in the CTNA feedback session is to outline the goals and structure of the feedback session to set the agenda or develop the contract with the patient. Developing the contract is important so that the session is a democratic process that does not flounder and become unstructured. A democratic process is one where there is circumscribed freedom of therapeutic dialogue. This means that the overarching framework is one where the patient will receive information from the results of the tests, but within that framework, the patient is free to comment on, question, and agree or disagree with results. In addition, the patient is free to comment on how they see the results applying to their life and functioning and to develop their own ideas as to how they would like to use the test results. In order to develop the "spirit" of this framework, the CTNA clinician may want to open the session with the following statement:

"I want to thank you for your willingness to attend this session and with your permission I'd like to begin by giving you an idea how the session will progress, would that be all right with you? [*Patient gives permission*]. I will give you the results from the tests you took previously. However, this session will not just be me giving you information; I hope it will be a dialogue between the two of us. I will be going over what is called a personal feedback report. This report includes your scores on each of the tests that you took and whether the skill that test assesses is a strength or weakness for you. I will review each test with you and make sure that you understand what the results mean. I want you to feel free to ask questions, make comments, agree or disagree with results. But what is most important is that we work together to find out how these results apply to your life and to any problems you might be experiencing related to the issues you presented with. In doing so I hope we can use these results to develop plans and goals for helping you improve life areas that you are concerned about. How does all that sound to you?"

The clinician should then invite the patient to ask any questions or make any comments. The clinician should answer any questions directly and clarify any misconceptions about what the test results will show or how the session will progress. Experience suggests that many patients find neuropsychological assessments interesting and challenging and are highly inquisitive about their performance. However, there may be performance anxieties as patients are often concerned about their cognitive abilities. They may have noticed difficulties with memory, attention, concentration, or other skills. Thus, it is a good idea to spend a few minutes providing empathy and support and clarifying any misconceptions or concerns patients have about receiving personal feedback about their cognitive abilities.

Check-In

Before beginning the actual feedback process, it is often helpful to provide a check-in to assess how the patient's life has been since the initial assessment. It is important to note any changes, new developments, setbacks, or successes. In addition to developing rapport, this helps to gain information that may lead to modifications of the test interpretations.

As part of the check-in, it may be helpful to remind the patient of the CCEC as a means of organizing the information to be discussed. An example of a reminding statement may be as follows:

Clinician: "Now as I understood during our previous meeting(s), it seems that the main reason you came for this evaluation was because you want to go back to college (W), but feel as though there has always been a reason that completing work on time has been so difficult (CR). This difficulty has been really frustrating for you over the years and has even left you feeling down on yourself (ER). You hope that this evaluation could help you answer some questions about yourself such as whether or not you have a learning disability, ADHD, or some other problem that causes you to feel as though you work slowly compared to others. Is all that about right?"

Following a process of patient reactions, the clinician will provide the patient a copy of the feedback report and orient the patient to the paperwork.

A discussion of patient questions or concerns about the feedback process easily flows into an explanation of the purpose for providing neuropsychological test feedback. Patients often have misconceptions about what it means to receive cognitive test feedback. Examples of patient misconceptions include the following:

- "You're going to tell me if I have brain damage."
- "You're going to tell me if I have Alzheimer's."
- "You're going to tell me if I'm crazy."
- "You're going to tell me how to solve Brian's problems."

The clinician will clarify for the patient that the purpose of the report is to provide the following: (1) an assessment of cognitive strengths and weaknesses; (2) the relationship between the tests results, the skills assessed, daily life problems, and behaviors that are of concern; and (3) ways to use the test results to develop more applicable and realistic treatment goals that address life areas of concern to the patient.

Next, the clinician will ask the patient about their recollection of taking the neuropsychological assessment and what general reactions they had. Neuropsychological testing is likely to be new for patients, and experience suggests that they may have reactions to the testing itself. This is because the skills required to complete these tests may relate to patients' functional performance in life areas of concern. As a result, patients may have thoughts and feelings triggered from the test stimulus, and the clinician should provide an opportunity to discuss these reactions. This process is important because patients will begin to see the feedback session as a collaborative endeavor where the patient and clinician work together to explore what the test results mean for the individual. For example, a patient may initially state that the test results stimulated concerns about their memory. However, through further exploration, it may be that memory concerns are part of a larger concern, which the patient is beginning to notice a significant change between who they used to be and who they are now. This may trigger feelings of sadness and loss. The following scenario demonstrates this.

Clinician: Ok, this part of the report talks about what neuropsychological assessment is. So let me ask you this, you took these yesterday, do you remember taking them yesterday? [Providing information and closed-ended question assessing patient's recollection]

Patient: Yes

Clinician: Tell me, what was it like for you taking all those tests? [Open-ended question]

Patient: It made me see where my thinking is at. It made me think about my memory and some things my memory is good on and some things my memory is not.... I think I have a blockage or something.... 'cause I will go upstairs and I know what I want ... before I get upstairs and I know what I'm going up there to get but when I get there I can't remember.

Clinician: Ok, sounds like you notice you forget things but then you will remember them at some point and it's like they've blocked out of your mind for awhile, or like something keeps them from getting past a certain point .... [Reflective summary]

Patient: Right! Right! Exactly! That's scary.

The patient continued along this discussion by remembering times when they had severe memory lapses that often led to scary and dangerous consequences. The patient became visibly concerned during the session and, as it progressed, became sad because prior to the problematic event, the patient was a competent and mentally sharp professional. The change they saw created a psychological discrepancy in regard to how they would like to be versus how they are. This particular patient was very pleased to be a part of the feedback because they had been concerned about their memory for some time.

At this time, it is important for the clinician to interact with the patient in an MI-consistent manner using *OARS* based on MI principles. This helps the patient feel understood in their perceptions and gently leads them to begin exploring life areas of concern that may provide material for the next section of the feedback form, life implications.

Summary Points for Setting the Agenda and Introducing the Feedback Report

- Develop a "democratic" contract that includes providing cognitive information while creating an atmosphere of openness, acceptance, trust, and warmth in order to facilitate patient self-disclosure. Questions, comments, and inquiries about the tests and results are welcomed and encouraged.
- Discuss and clarify any patient questions or concerns about the feedback process in general.
- Provide a copy of a feedback report.
- Discuss the purpose of the feedback process as providing information about cognitive strengths and weaknesses, relating these areas to important life areas, and developing applicable and realistic treatment goals. Remind the patient of the CCEC as a means for organizing and structuring the feedback process.
- Discuss the patient's recollection of the testing process as a way to personalize the experience and enhance collaboration.
- Always interact with the patient in a person-centered manner using the MI strategies reflected in the acronym OARS.

Summary of the MI Verbal Skills "OARS" (Miller & Rollnick, 1991, 2002)

Open-ended question: Any question that requires elaboration versus one that can be answered with "yes" or "no."

Example: "Tell me about your medical history." *versus* "Do you have any medical problems?"

Affirmation: Affirming a patient's efforts at changing or understanding the need for change.

Example: "I really appreciate how you're struggling to understand this with me."

Reflection: An expression of empathy for something the patient said.

Example: "You're feeling angry because of the loss of your cognitive abilities."

Summary: A clinician's summarization of main points discussed in a session.

Example: "So what I've heard so far is that you've noticed a change in your ability to remember things; this has created quite a bit of distress for you and your family and as a result you're feeling like your role has changed completely, and this frightens you."

Step 2: Develop Life Implications Questions

In order to make the feedback report as useful as possible, patients provide specific questions they hope the test results will answer for them. Initial questions patients have are likely to be rather vague and nonspecific. Therefore, it helps the clinician to use MI skills in order to reflect, question, and elaborate on patient concerns so that the true nature of the question is brought about. An example of a vague concern a patient had was the following:

"Why do I keep relapsing into drug use?"

Through guidance and exploration, asking open-ended questions, and reflecting important themes and feelings, the clinician was able to develop a more specific question that the test results may be able to answer.

"Why am I not able to stay focused and organize my thoughts, which have led me to begin slipping in my recovery plan and eventually lead to relapse?"

Experience suggests that it is best to limit the life implications section to two or three well-developed questions. Too many questions are unlikely to be addressed in a 1-hour feedback report. It is also important to remind patients that test results are not guaranteed to answer all their questions. It may be that different types of tests, such as personality assessments, are more appropriate for some of their questions. However, experience suggests that the neuropsychological tests can provide guidance and direction to many questions patients have and in many cases provide concrete answers to specific concerns. For example, a patient in her mid-40s had concerns that she may have brain damage or early Alzheimer's disease as a result of her drug and alcohol usage. She had been abstinent for many months, but her memory did not seem to be improving. In a review of her test results, she scored in the high average and in some cases superior range on most tests of memory, but was in the low-average range on many tests of attention, concentration, and working memory. When the patient was given this feedback, and asked how it may have applied to her daily life, she began disclosing her frustrations with getting her life back together in early recovery. Although she felt better being clean and sober, she admitted that many areas of her life needed attention, including family, work, daily household tasks, in addition to debt she had accrued. She tried to go about life like everything was in order, but in reality, her mind was constantly racing with all these responsibilities, and she felt overwhelmed, disorganized, and unfocused. She had been afraid to tell anyone of her struggles because she was afraid they would just tell her to be patient and take one day at a time or that they might think she was on the verge of relapse if she told them how overwhelmed and depressed she felt.

After spending time listening to her thoughts and concerns and providing empathic support, the clinician asked permission to offer the patient some thoughts. The patient emphatically said "yes" and that any suggestions would be appreciated. The clinician suggested that, in fact, her memory is quite good but that her ability to attend to, organize, and carry out all the multiple, competing tasks has become overwhelming for her. As a result, she feels depressed, stressed, and inadequate, which further compromises her ability to attend to and organize all the many difficult and competing demands in her life. Although her drug use may have compromised some of these skills, it appears as though her depression and stress are more pronounced and have a greater affect on her.

The patient agreed with this and began to say how she has tried to ignore her depression and stress because she thought it meant she was weak and not following a good recovery program. After further discussion and exploration, the clinician and patient agreed on a change plan that consisted of (1) using cognitive–behavioral strategies to organize and prioritize her multiple competing demands while challenging negative thoughts about her competency and self-worth; (2) working on reducing her stress and depression by taking time for herself; (3) considering a medication regimen; and (4) working more closely with her primary clinician on these particular issues and reducing the shame associated with them.

This is an example of how neuropsychological tests and feedback can provide a bridge between cognitive and emotional issues while potentially answering salient life concerns.

The introduction to the feedback report is not merely a quick description of the feedback in order to lead in to the rest of the report. The introduction phase begins the development of a collaborative relationship where the clinician and the patient are working together to discover what the neuropsychological test results mean to the individual. By the end of the introductory session, the clinician will have elicited from the patient what life areas are of most concern for them and how the cognitive test results can potentially answer important questions that patients have about their lives and their ability to function.

Summary Points for Developing Life Implications Questions

- Use clinical skills to develop questions into well-developed and specific questions that provide guidance for the CTNA feedback session.
- Limit the number of questions to two or three. Too few questions are likely to leave the patient feeling unfinished. Too many questions are unlikely to be addressed and also may leave the patient feeling unfinished.
- Acknowledge the strengths and limitations of testing by helping patients understand that not all questions can be answered by neuropsychological tests.
- Consistently interact with the patient in a person-centered manner, using OARS to reflect and clarify the nature of patient questions and concerns.

Step 3: Determining a Personal Skill Profile

In the next phase of a feedback session, a clinician provides information on how a skill is rated as a personal strength or weakness. Our experience is that it is best to keep such an analysis simple and straightforward. Therefore, we have three categories: above average, average, and below average. To determine where an individual's score falls, we convert the raw score into a percentile.

A percentile is a standard measure of how an individual's raw test score is compared to other individuals who have taken the same test. For example, if an individual's score falls in the 25th percentile, this means that this individual scored better than 24% of those who have taken the test and worse than 74% of those who have taken the test. On the contrary, if an individual's score falls in the 80th percentile, it means that this person scored better than 79% of people who have taken the same test and worse than 19% of people who have taken the same test.

An individual's test is considered in the below-average range when their score falls in the 24th percentile or less. An individual's score is considered to be in the average range if their score falls between the 25th and 75th percentiles. A score is in the above-average range if it falls in the 76th percentile or greater.

It is important that the clinicians use whatever measurement that best suits them. The scale of measurement identified above was used in the NAFI study because it was felt that this would be most understandable to the patient group. It is important that the scale of measurement is understandable to the patient and that they understand how this scale was developed. This requires an open conversation about norm-based scoring, how scores are derived, and the strengths and limitations of this type of scoring. A second important factor is that patients should understand that norm-based scoring is a method for describing their cognitive functioning in relation to peers who are similar to them. However, the scoring does not presume to describe *who the patient is as a person*. Norm-based scores are tools that serve to describe one piece of a patients' world, not the patient as a whole person.

Summarizing How a Personal Skill Profile Is Determined

- Explain that a skill is rated in one of three ways: average, above average, or below average.
- Average scores are scores that fall between the 25th and 75th percentiles, above-average scores are above the 75th percentile, and below-average scores are lower than the 25th percentile.
- Use a graphic illustration to explain the concept to patients (see example below).

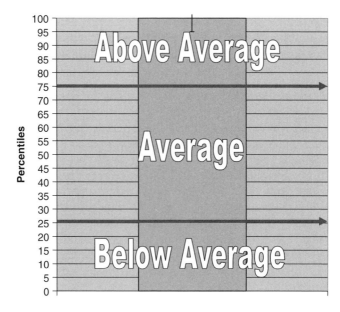

Figure 5.1 Example graph from the NAFI Personal Feedback Report from the study Effects of Cognitive Test Feedback on Patient Adherence

Step 4: Individual Test Results: Feedback About Personal Strengths and Weaknesses

The following section will describe the procedures for providing feedback from individual test results. The general conceptual framework for providing feedback will be described in addition to case examples.

The section has three main purposes: (1) to provide patients information about functional strengths that they have based on neuropsychological test results, (2) to identify the relationship between cognitive strengths and daily life concerns, and (3) to identify ways patients' personal strengths can be used to aid in resolving life problems.

Introducing the test and the skills examined

The first step of the feedback process is for the clinician to (a) briefly describe the nature of the test being discussed and elicit from the patient (b) what memories they have about taking the test and (c) what skills *they* saw the test as examining. This is important so that the patient is an active participant in the feedback process and is able to express what the experience meant to them. An example of an introductory statement includes the following:

"This test is called the Wisconsin Card Sorting Test. This is the test you took on the computer where you had to match cards to a series of key cards and were given feedback as to whether you were right or wrong. Do you remember taking this test?"

Examples of probing open-ended questions are as follows

- Can you tell me what it was like for you to take this test?
- What skills did you seem yourself as having to use in order to effectively complete this test?
- In what way(s) do you use these skills in your daily life?
- How do you think these skills are working for you in your daily life?
- In what way(s) do these skills have an impact on your [injury or illness]?

Mental skills are addressed in this way so that the patient can put the cognitive abilities in their own words and then relate these skills to their daily life, problems, and concerns. Even if the patient does not precisely state what skills the tests measure, it is more important to have the patient think about the nature of the tests and the meaning(s) derived from them. In this way, the testing experience becomes more personal and applicable to the patient's life.

When working with children and adolescents, feedback is often provided primarily to parents or other caregivers. In these situations, it is often helpful to describe a test by showing parents the testing materials so that they might fully understand the nature of their child's performance. For example, many parents can quickly surmise the challenges in copying the Rey figure and completing block design or matrix reasoning. It can be helpful to have parents respond to a few example questions when introducing tests such as vocabulary, information, or similarities.

"Elicit–Provide–Elicit" and OARS

When providing information about cognitive tests, CTNA follows the framework of "Elicit–Provide–Elicit" from MI. When beginning the process of providing information, the clinician first *elicits* reactions from the patient about the test itself and their perceptions of what skills they saw themselves as using and how they think they performed. This serves to personalize the test results for the patient and enhance the collaborative nature of the feedback process. Second, the clinician asks permission to *provide* information about the nature of the tests, the skills they assess, and ways these skills are used in daily life. Asking permission is a key concept in the provision of information in MI. The clinician asks permission because the goal is to empower the patient to accept or reject the information as applying to them. This also avoids the "expert trap" where information is imparted in a top-down manner, with the patient being a passive recipient of the clinician's "expertise". When addressed in this manner, the majority of patients will give permission to the clinician to provide information. Once the clinician provides information, the next step is to *elicit* patient reactions to the information. This allows the patient to comment on the applicability and usefulness of the information to their daily lives and concerns.

Throughout the introduction and eliciting of patient reactions, it is important for the clinician to go back to using OARS. The goal is to clarify patient reactions to the testing experience and what the experience meant to the patient in terms of stimulating ideas about how they see themselves functioning and finally to enhance the patient's ability to apply the tests and what they measure to their daily life. Patients may be able to express vague knowledge of the connection between test results and their daily lives. However, skillful reflective listening and evocative, open-ended questions can further develop the applicability of the test results to patient life problems and concerns. The following sections will illustrate this process more in depth.

Providing Information from the Test Results

Once the clinician has elicited information from the patient and used OARS to clarify the patient's perceptions, the clinician may then provide information to the patient about the skills an individual test assesses. The important task here is not to use fancy words or jargon in describing the cognitive skills. The feedback report provides bulleted descriptions of each cognitive skill in simple layman's terms. Table 5.1 provides the cognitive terms along with more simplistic, layman definitions.

Table 5.1

Neuropsychological term	Layman definition
Executive functioning	Analyze and solve problems, identify patterns, make correct decisions, hold ideas in your head, organize and sequence plans, be flexible in your thinking, solve a problem logically, focus without getting distracted
Attention and concentration	Pay attention and remember things, hold ideas in your head and reverse them, focus, concentrate
Learning and memory	Remember words or stories that are read to you, recover memories from things told to you a long time ago,
Motor skills	Work quickly with your hands and fingers
Visuospatial ability	Accurately copy things you see

Elicit Patient Reactions to the Information

Once the clinician has provided the patient information about the cognitive skills, the next step is to again *elicit* from the patient their reactions to hearing the cognitive skills as a strength and in what areas of their life they see the skill operating. The clinician then uses *OARS* in order to reflect and clarify the patient's perception of how they see this skill operating in their life and what it means to them. Some important questions a clinician might pose to the patient include the following:

- "How do you see yourself using these skills in your daily life?"
- "How does these skills relate to some of the questions you posed at the beginning of the session?"
- "Can you see how this skill might be a problem for your daughter?"
- "What relationship do you see to these skills and issues related to your [presenting problem]?"

The purpose of such questions is to facilitate patient self-disclosure and open a dialogue as to how the test results apply to patient real-world problems and concerns.

Example #1 The following example provides a segment of a session where the patient is given information about a cognitive skill determined to be a personal strength:

A patient receiving feedback had performed within the average range on the Wisconsin Card Sorting Test. A graphical illustration (Fig. 5.2) of the results appears as follows:

The results indicated that the patient performed within the average range in regard to the number of categories achieved (6/6), number of errors (48th percentile), and perseverative errors made (38th percentile). Based on these results the following conversation ensued:

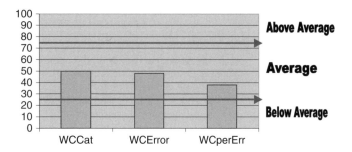

Figure 5.2 Graphical illustration of a patient's performance on the Wisconsin Card Sorting Test

Clinician: Ok, let's go over this test here called the Wisconsin Card Sorting Test. That's the test you did on the computer where you had to match different cards to four key cards on the top of the screen. [Providing information]

Do you remember having taken this test? [Closed question]

Patient: Yes.

Clinician: What do you remember about that test? [Elicits patient reactions to the test with an open-ended question]

Patient: It was really challenging. (laughs) I remember looking at it, trying to see what way it was supposed to go, and then once I thought I got it, it would be wrong so I had to figure out another way.

Clinician: It was a curious and confusing test because it shifted on you. [Amplified reflection]

Patient: Yeah, first it would be blue circles, then red triangles, then red circles, and it just kept changing and changing.

Clinician: So you really had to be on your toes. [Simple reflection]

What was it like for you to have to do that? [Open-ended question]

Patient: I liked that! I could play that every day!

Clinician: So you really enjoyed that. [Simple reflection]

What was it that was most enjoyable for you? [Open-ended question]

Patient: Just the challenge, analyzing things, having to figure it out. I've always liked those kinds of things because that's what I did when I used to work. I had to analyze problems and find solutions to things.

Clinician: So this test really tapped into something you like to do and in fact are enthusiastic about. [Amplified reflection]

Would you like to know what this tests measures and how you did? [Closed-ended question asking permission to give information]

Patient: Yeah, absolutely.

Clinician: This test assesses a lot of what you just mentioned, your ability to analyze and solve problems, to figure out patterns to things, and to benefit from feedback about your performance so you can change something that might not be going well. [Providing information]

According to the results, you performed in the average range on this test, which means you did as well as anyone else who has taken this. [Providing information]

What are your thoughts about how that fits for you and your life? [Elicits patient reaction to the information with an open-ended question]

Patient: (Pauses) I think that's how I've survived all these years.

Clinician: Really? Tell me about that. [Open-ended question]

Patient: That's how I survived. I've been through a lot and there are times I wasn't sure I was going to make it. There are other times when I look back and I think that I should be dead. But somehow, I've been able to look at where I am and once I realize what it is I need to do, I try to set things in motion so that I'm around positive people and positive things. It isn't always easy but as many times as I've fallen down, I've picked myself back up.

Clinician: You're a survivor. [Amplified reflection]

Patient: (Pauses, smiles) I guess I am. Yeah, you're right, I am.

The above scenario demonstrates how the test results are used to create a bridge between the patient's cognitive abilities and important life issues. The patient's performance on the Wisconsin Card Sorting Test is an illustration of how they have used their analytical skills to survive in very difficult times. This information can be used later when the clinician and the patient work together to develop strategies for resolving important life issues the patient is struggling with. Furthermore, the clinician and patient collaborate to discover the patient's personal resources for resolving problems in their life. This will be important when discussing ways to adapt or cope with weaknesses.

Example #2 In this scenario, a clinician is providing feedback to the mother of an 8-year-old boy who is having behavior problems in school. He was referred for the evaluation of a learning disability versus attention-deficit/hyperactivity disorder. The test results indicate that his behavior problems are likely the result of undiagnosed dyslexia and that he displays no cognitive markers of attention problems. The following is an example of the dialogue between the parent and the clinician.

Clinician: The first test I want to talk about is called the Continuous Performance Test. Jason took this test on a computer in my office. [Providing information]

Did he tell you about it? [Closed-ended question]

Parent: I don't think so.

Clinician: Ok, on this test, he had to look at the computer screen while different random letters are flashed on the screen, one at a time. Sometimes they go fast, other times they go more slowly. Each time that he saw a letter, he had to press the space bar – except when he saw the letter X. When he saw the letter X, he had to try not to hit the space bar. One trick here is that the test takes sort of a long time – around 12 or 15 minutes. [Providing information]

   What do you think this test was getting at? [Open-ended question]

Parent: Well, it seems really boring. I'm guessing that he'd need to pay attention to this boring game for a long period of time. And he'd have to try real hard to not react when he's not supposed to.

Clinician: Exactly right! The test is a great measure of one type of attention and ability to not be impulsive. [Providing information]

   Can you think of how this skill might be useful in Jason's life? [Open-ended question]

Parent: Well, it's a lot like school. He's gotta sit there all day and pay attention to things that maybe aren't as interesting as his video games.

Clinician: Bingo! In order for him to be successful in school, he needs to be able to sit there and filter out the junk and focus on the important stuff. [Amplified reflection]

   So, how do you think he did? [Elicit]

Parent: Oh, I'm afraid that he probably bombed it. I imagine that he hit that space bar for nearly everything, but eventually, he just quit or got frustrated.

Clinician: Well, would you like for me to tell you about his scores? [Closed-ended question asking permission to give information]

Parent: Yeah, although I'm not sure I want to know (laughs).

Clinician: Jason performed in the high average range on this test. His score showed no impulsivity or distractibility throughout the entire process. It's exactly what we would expect, or better, from other eight year-old boys. [Providing information]

   What do you think about that? [Elicits parent reaction to the information with an open-ended question]

Parent: I'm totally surprised. Are you sure you scored that correctly (laughs)? So, this test of attention didn't show that Jason has trouble?

Clinician: No. In fact, he did rather well. You look a little stunned. [Reflection]

Parent: Yeah, it's just so different from what I would expect.

From this point, the clinician and parent went on to discuss the weaknesses noted on measures of lexical processing and phonemic decoding that underlie Jason's learning disability. Like all neuropsychological assessment, CTNA assessment can help patients and their families revisit personal narratives and ways of understanding problematic behavior. However, CTNA offers patients and families a voice in the process so that the new narrative is their own.

Summarizing the Provision of Individual Test Results: Strengths

- Introduce each test by first eliciting memories from the patient about the test itself and what skills they saw themselves as using to complete the test.
- Ask the patient for permission to provide information about the skills individual tests assess.
- Use the Elicit–Provide–Elicit framework from MI when providing neuro-psychological test information:

  - Elicit patient reactions and memories about the tests.
  - Provide information about the tests and the skills they assess.
  - Elicit patient reactions to the information provided.

- When providing neuropsychological test information, avoid jargon and discuss the cognitive skills in simple, layman's terms using examples where appropriate.
- When eliciting patient reactions, use OARS to reflect and clarify patient thoughts and perceptions.

Feedback About Difficulties or Weaknesses

Providing feedback about cognitive difficulties or weaknesses follows the same basic format as for personal strengths with similar goals: (1) to provide patients information about functional weaknesses based on neuropsychological test results, (2) to identify the relationship between cognitive weaknesses and daily life concerns, and (3) to identify ways cognitive weaknesses may be contributing to life problems and ways to adapt, cope with, or possibly remediate these weaknesses.

Introducing the Test and the Skills Examined

Providing patients information about cognitive weaknesses follows the same format as those for personal strengths. The clinician first *elicits* memories that patients have about taking the test and then uses *OARS* to reflect, clarify, and understand the patient's perception of what skills they used and how they see these skills applying to their daily life.

Providing Information About Cognitive Weaknesses

The clinician now may *provide* information to the patient about the cognitive weaknesses and what skills the test assesses. Providing this information requires sensitivity on the part of the clinician to pay attention to patient reactions.

Experience suggests that most patients are able to deal well with hearing that they have cognitive weaknesses, although there are times when patients may jump to conclusions and think that a cognitive weakness has some catastrophic meaning. There is also the possibility that a patient's cognitive profile may suggest more serious problems. Such issues will be discussed in the section on special issues.

Elicit Patient Reactions to the Information

The clinician will now *elicit* patient reactions to hearing information about cognitive weaknesses and what areas of their life they see the skill operating. The clinician then uses OARS in order to reflect and clarify the patient's perception of how they see these skills operating in their life and what it means to them. It is during this process that patients may express some form of resistance to the test results, and it is important that the clinician respond to patient resistance in a manner consistent with the person-centered principles of MI.

The following example demonstrates providing information about cognitive weaknesses.

Clinician: Janet we're going to shift now and discuss test results that you struggled with or are what we call weaknesses. [Providing information] Are you ready to discuss these? [Closed-ended question assessing Janet's readiness to review these areas]

Patient: Yeah, I think so.

Clinician: Ok, let's look at this first test called Letter Number Sequencing. This was the test where I read to you a series of numbers and letters and you had to put them all in the right order, numbers first and then the letters. [Providing information] Do you remember this test? [Closed-ended question]

Patient: Oh, yeah, that was hard.

Clinician: Tell me what it was like for you while taking that test. [Open-ended question]

Patient: I remember that one being really confusing. The first two were ok but after that there were just too many numbers and letters and I just got lost.

Clinician: So it became a bit overwhelming for you. [Simple reflection] What kind of things did you have to do in order to complete this test? [Open-ended question]

Patient: Well, I had to pay real close attention to what you were saying and try to remember what you said when you read another set of numbers or letters. That's what became frustrating, is when I thought you were done reading some numbers you started with another set of letters and I couldn't remember what you previously said.

Clinician: It sounds like you really tried to hold on to what was told to you but it became too much and the old information gave way to the new. [Amplified reflection]

Patient: Yeah, something like that, I could only remember so much.

Clinician: Ok, well can I tell you what we know this test to assess. [Closed - ended question asking permission]

Patient: Yes, mmm hmm.

Clinician: You're pretty much on the mark with what you noticed this test to assess. This test measures what we call "working memory". This is your ability to hold pieces of information in your head for a period of time and then do something with that information. [Providing information]

Patient: Kind of like adding numbers in your head?

Clinician: Yes very much like that. You have to hold different thoughts in your mind and then use that information in some way. It's kind of like if your clinician tells you to go to a 12-step meeting, get a sponsor, take some literature, get a signature from the chairman, and meet at least three people. You use your working memory to hold all those different ideas in your head and then figure out how you're going to do all that. Does that make sense? [Providing information/closed-ended question assessing comprehension]

Patient: Oh, yeah. I have a big problem with that. Whenever I set out to do something that is kind of complicated, I almost always forget some part of it.

Clinician: Ok, well in fact the test shows that you do struggle with this. Your score fell in the low average range, or 16th percentile. It sounds like you recognize this is a problem can you tell me more about that? [Providing information/elicit patient reactions with an open-ended question]

Patient: Just like in group. I can't remember everything they talk about. I hear what's being said and I'm trying to pay attention to it, but then they keep going on and I'm still stuck on the previous topic and I completely miss what's being said.

Clinician: Do you think it matters what the topic of conversation is? [Closed-ended question]

Patient: No, I don't think so. Because it happens all the time. I go out to smoke break and everyone is talking about the group and I don't remember at least half of what was talked about. So eventually I just say to hell with it.

Clinician: It sounds like you're worried you might be missing some important things. [Amplified reflection]

Patient: I know I am. People think I just don't care or I'm not paying attention. I'm trying but I just can't focus on all that stuff at one time.

In the above example, the patient has been experiencing difficulties with working memory that were interpreted as lack of motivation. Providing concrete feedback in an understandable way created insight that was useful to the patient and explained something they had been struggling with.

Summarizing the Provision of Individual Test Results: Weaknesses

- Introduce each test by first eliciting memories from the patient about the test itself and what skills they saw themselves as using to complete the test.
- Ask the patient for permission to provide information about the skills individual tests assess.
- Use the Elicit–Provide–Elicit framework from MI when providing neuro-psychological test information:
  - Elicit patient reactions and memories about the tests.
  - Provide information about the tests and the skills they assess.
  - Elicit patient reactions to the information provided.
- When providing neuropsychological test information, avoid jargon and discuss the cognitive skills in simple, layman's terms using examples where appropriate.
- When eliciting patient reactions, use OARS to reflect and clarify patient thoughts and perceptions.

Responding to Resistance

It is possible that, when presenting cognitive weaknesses, patients may be resistant to hearing such information due to shock or fear or because the results seem discrepant from their own experience. If this happens, it is important that clinicians follow the MI principle of "rolling with resistance." In MI, resistance is not challenged directly but met with understanding, empathy, and openness by the clinician to empathize with the patient's perception of the situation.

In MI, there are two sets of strategies for responding to patient resistance reflective and strategic approaches. Reflective approaches are statements made by the clinician that empathizes with a patient's perception of a situation. Reflective statements are simple yet are often effective means of disarming resistant dialogue and guiding the conversation to a more therapeutic topic. Miller and Rollnick (1991, 2002) identify five different types of reflective statements.

1. *Simple reflection*: The clinician says back to the patient what they just said, staying close to his or her words.

Patient: Are you sure these tests are right? I've never noticed this kind of problem before.
Clinician: You're wondering of the tests are accurate.

2. *Reflection of feeling*: The clinician reflects back to the patient the underlying affect expressed in their statement.

Patient: (Eyes wide open, wringing their hands) I can't believe I performed so poorly on this test!

Clinician: You're rather shocked by this and feeling very nervous about what this might mean.

3. *Reflection of meaning*: The clinician reflects the implied cognitive content of what the patient says.

Patient: I'm a little nervous about hearing the results given that my father had dementia when he was near my age.

Clinician: Your worried what these results might mean for your future and what could happen to you.

4. *Double-sided reflection*: The clinician reflects both sides of a conflict the patient may express.

Patient: Yes, my wife has told me I don't seem as sharp as I used to be but I think she may just be over-reacting.

Clinician: You're not really worried about your faculties but other people have expressed concern.

5. **Amplified reflection**: It is used when the patient has expressed only the negative side of a conflict: The clinician intensifies what the patient has said, which usually leads the patient to correct the distortion. For example:

Patient: Yes I forget things now and then but doesn't everyone my age?

Clinician: It seems like your memory is just as good as everyone else you know and there appears to be no reason for concern.

Often clinicians may use strategic approaches to handle resistant statements. Examples of strategic approaches include shifting focus to another topic with the hopes of coming back to the more emotionally charged topic, reframing a statement, emphasizing patients' personal choice and control, and paradoxical interventions (Miller and Rollnick, 1991, 2002). Examples of these strategies are as follows:

1. *Shifting focus*: This refers to the clinician shifting away from an emotionally charged topic to one that engenders less resistance with the hopes of coming back at a later time.

Patient: I think the test is wrong! There is no way my concentration could be that poor!

Clinician: So you see you're ability to focus and concentrate as pretty good. What kind of things have you noticed that tells you that?

2. *Reframe*: This refers to presenting what the patient has said from a different perspective.

Patient: I don't see why my mother should take this medication if it's not going to stop her from becoming demented.
Clinician: You really only want something if you think it's going to cure her.

3. *Emphasizing personal choice and control*: This assures the patient that whether they take any action or not is completely in their hands.

Patient: I've already been to speech, occupational and physical therapy, I don't want to go to something else, I'm tired of all this therapy and I still can't think through things the way I used to.
Clinician: Although I believe that this rehabilitation program could help you, you are right that it is totally your choice and I understand that this has been a long hard road.

4. *Paradoxical intervention*: This is a last resort intervention. It refers to the clinician "coming alongside" the patient's perception and agreeing with them as a way to disarm the resistance and bring the patient to a more balanced view. This must be done with sincerity and sensitivity so as not to seem sarcastic.

Patient: My doctor told me that I have severe damage to my brain, so if that's the case then nothing can be done and I'm not going to any more programs just to spin my wheels.
Clinician: I can see that you think nothing else can be done and you sound pretty set that you're not interested in doing any more therapy. Perhaps you're right that this isn't the right time to think about any further treatment. Would it be all right if I just shared a few thoughts with you anyway?

In providing neuropsychological results, a clinician deals with resistance by (1) rolling with it as is consistent with MI principles, (2) acknowledging the strengths and weaknesses of neuropsychological tests, and (3) ensuring that the relationship between test skills and actual real-life functional behavior has been adequately illustrated.

1. Rolling with resistance: The first step in rolling with resistance is to recognize that resistance is occurring. Resistance usually takes the form of four types of behaviors: when a patient openly argues with the clinician about test results, interrupts the clinician during an explanation, negates information the clinician provides, or outright ignores the clinician (Miller & Rollnick, 1991, 2002). In providing neuropsychological information, such behaviors are likely to occur if the information provided is discrepant from the patient's own viewpoint or if the information upsets the patient for any number of reasons. Should this occur, clinician's responses to the patient that are not helpful include the following: arguing that the test results are correct, assuming an expert role, criticizing or belittling the patient in some way, labeling the patient as being in denial or resistant, or stating that the test results hold some preeminence over the patient's viewpoint. The following scenario demonstrates a poor way to handle resistance in the CTNA.

Clinician: James, the results of the test you took called the Logical Memory Test indicates that you have some problems with your memory.

Patient: Really? I thought I did well on that?

Clinician: No, actually you scored in the 5th percentile, which is considered in the borderline range.

Patient: What does that mean?

Clinician: It means you're almost in the impaired range but not quite.

Patient: I just don't see how that can be, I thought my memory was pretty good.

Clinician: No it's quite low. Perhaps your alcohol use has caused some memory problems. Research suggests that even social drinkers can have some problems with memory but your level of drinking places you in a more severe category. Therefore it would be expected that your memory would be more impaired.

Patient: Wait, wait, slow down. I don't see my memory as impaired. I think I remember stuff pretty good, I'm not sure where you're getting this stuff.

Clinician: These tests are highly reliable estimations of cognition. The Logical Memory test has shown to have a reliability estimate of between 0.7 and 0.9, which means that it's very good at picking up memory problems. I really think you need to consider this.

Patient: Well I don't care what or who it relies on. I'm saying it's wrong, I've never noticed a problem with my memory.

Clinician: What has your wife said?

Patient: About what? What's she got to do with this?!

Clinician: I can see this has upset you but the fact of the matter is you're showing memory problems and we need to talk about what can be done about that. Shall we move on?

Patient: Yeah, right.

The following is the same scenario with the clinician responding to the patient in a more MI consistent fashion.

Clinician: James, do you remember the test where stories were read to you and you had to remember them? What was that like for you? [Open-ended question assessing comprehension and memory of the test]

Patient: That was fine, I think I did pretty well on that.

Clinician: Ok, so trying to remember those stories was not a problem. [Simple reflection] How does that apply to your ability to remember things on a day to day basis? [Open-ended question]

Patient: It's ok as far as I can tell. I've never had a problem with it.

Clinician: Ok, well would you like to see how the test results turned out? [Closed-ended question asking permission to provide information]

Patient:	Yeah.
Clinician:	According to the results, your score on the first logical memory test, which is a test of short term memory or your ability to remember the story after a short period of time, your score fell in the 5th percentile. [Providing information] What thoughts do you have about that? [Open-ended question]
Patient:	What does that mean?
Clinician:	That means that you scored higher than about 4% of people who have taken this test and lower than 94% of people who have taken this test. We would say that score falls in the borderline range, which is not impaired, but lower than below average. [Providing information] How does that fit for you and how you saw your performance? [Open-ended question]
Patient:	That can't be right!
Clinician:	You're surprised by this? [Simple reflection of affect]
Patient:	Yeah, I thought I did good. I can't believe you're saying my memory is that bad.
Clinician:	So this is really concerning to you and doesn't fit with the way you see yourself remembering things on a daily basis. [Amplified reflection]
Patient:	Well, yeah, I mean…I just don't see my memory as that bad.
Clinician:	This seems upsetting to you. [Simple reflection]
Patient:	Yeah, I mean, I don't see it as *this* bad anyway.
Clinician:	So it doesn't seem like it should be as bad as this but now that you think of it there might be some things you've noticed that concern you. [Double-sided reflection]
Patient:	Well, I mean there are times when my wife has said that she told me something and I insist she didn't.
Clinician:	What kind of situations has that created? [Open-ended question]
Patient:	Well that's one of the things we fight about.

This scenario provides an example of rolling with patient resistance. In this case the patient questioned the validity of the test. Instead of becoming defensive and justifying, the clinician empathized and asked a few nonthreatening yet evocative open-ended questions, which lowered the patient's resistance enough to where he admitted that there may have been some discrepancy between how he sees himself versus how he really is. This leads into the next principle for dealing with resistance.

2. Acknowledging the strengths and weaknesses of neuropsychological tests. There is ample evidence to suggest that neuropsychological tests are valid estimations of functional behavior. However, as with all tests, neuropsychological tests have their limitations. For example, the conditions of the testing situation may affect performance. Conditions such as room temperature, lighting, rapport with the examiner, stress of the task, and patient variables such as how much sleep they had, if they had a meal, level of fatigue, and others all may affect how valid a test is in measuring a specific skill. Another example relates to the nature of specific tests. Neuropsychological tests are designed to measure specific cognitive skills; however, many tests actually measure a variety of different skills, and it may be difficult to discern which skill contributes to a poor score. The important concept is that neuropsychological tests are potentially valid and powerful measures of functional skill, but they are not perfect. Thus, one way to diffuse resistance and begin a dialogue to determine if a test score is valid is to simply acknowledge the strengths and weaknesses of cognitive tests.

Clinician: Ok, let's go onto the next test. Do you remember the test where you had to put pegs in holes as quickly as you can? [Closed-ended question] What was that like for you? [Open-ended question]

Patient: I really hated that one. My dexterity has never been good.

Clinician: Ok, so that really wasn't a good test for you and it sounds like it tested a skill you know yourself to struggle with. [Simple reflection]

Patient: Yeah I never was good with my hands.

Clinician: Ok, well would you like to know how you did? [Closed-ended question]

Patient: I can see here that I look pretty low but that doesn't surprise me.

Clinician: So this is not news for you, what have you noticed about your abilities in this area? [Open-ended question]

Patient: Well I've never had good eye-hand coordination, that's why I've never been good at things that I have to use my hands. So I think that's really all its testing.

Clinician: Ok, so this is something that's been around for a while. [Simple reflection] And in fact, you're right, this test does not really give information about whether your score is related to an actual problem due to substance use or whether this is just the way you are. [Providing information that affirms the patient] However, I would like to make one observation if you're willing to hear it? [Closed-ended question asking patients' permission to provide information]

Patient: Sure.

Clinician: Your score fell in what we would call the impaired range, meaning that more than 99% of people who took this test scored higher than you. This reminds me of the fact that you have been concerned about tingling in your arms and feet. [Providing information] What concerns do you have about that? [Open-ended question]

In this scenario, the clinician acknowledges the limitations of the test but then asks an open-ended and evocative question that lays the groundwork for placing doubt in the patient's mind that there really is no problem. The patient represented in this scenario did, in fact, have peripheral neuropathy possibly related to alcohol use.

3. Illuminating the relationship between test skills and functional behavior. Ideally, this concept should have already been made clear but may need to be revisited if the patient does not comprehend the connection. The clinician needs to make sure they have adequately elicited from the patient what skills they saw themselves using to complete a test and then express how they see those skills operating in their daily life. Second, cognitive skills should be described in simple, layman's terms with examples provided. Consider the following example of a patient who does not understand why they scored in the low-average range on the Wisconsin Card Sorting Test.

Patient: I couldn't understand that test; I don't think it was fair; I'm a good problem solver.

Clinician: So this doesn't fit with how you see yourself? [Reflection of meaning]

Patient: No, not at all. I'm good at puzzles and things and I play cards all the time so I can't understand it!

Clinician: Ok, I can see this is frustrating for you. [Simple reflection] Can we talk a bit about what specific things you had to do for this test? [Closed-ended question asking permission to provide information]

Patient: Yeah, ok.

Clinician: It seemed like early on in the test you had a hard time figuring out what you were being asked to do. You would figure out a pattern, get a few cards right and then suddenly switch. One of the things you have to do to complete this test is to focus and concentrate for an extended period of time and then wait for the test to tell you whether a move you made was right or wrong, and then use that feedback to figure out another pattern. It seemed though like you were trying to get ahead of the game. [Summary of clinician observations] How do you see that working in your regular life? [Open-ended question]

Patient: (Silent, thinking). You know what; I have been told that I'm impulsive.

Clinician: Really? Can you tell me more about that? [Open-ended question]

Patient: Yeah, y'know, sometimes I just go with things. I don't sit and think I just run with it and next thing y'know I'm in trouble.

Clinician: Do you think that might have been happening while taking this test? [Closed-ended question]

Patient: (Laughs) Yeah I think it was.

This example demonstrates how the patient was able to come to their own insight that inattentiveness and impulsiveness may be affecting their problem-solving and decision-making skills. What was needed was further clarification by the clinician as to what specific skills are assessed with the test and encouraging the patient to think of these skills in real-world terms.

Summary of Providing Skill Profiles

The important things to consider in providing information from neuropsychological tests in CTNA is that the clinician must first elicit answers from the patient in regard to how they saw their performance, what skills they see the test measuring, and how the skills related to the patient's daily life. At the same time, the clinician should be interacting with the patient in an MI-consistent manner using reflections and open-ended and evocative questions, affirming the patient, and summarizing thoughts. The clinician must emanate a spirit of collaboration with the patient or family, respect their autonomy as an individual, and continually evoke thoughts and reactions from the patient versus falling into a question-and-answer trap where the patient is merely a passive recipient. When the clinician offers information from the test results, s/he does so in a nonjudgmental and objective manner, always making sure the patient is ready to hear this information. Throughout the information provision, the clinician maintains an attitude of respect and unconditional regard and avoids labels or complicated cognitive jargon. Questions are answered directly and objectively, and patient reactions to the information is elicited and further empathized with and clarified. As such, the provision of feedback is not a one-sided, top-down endeavor where the clinician passively imparts information to the patient. The interaction is one of collaboration and equality where the clinician maintains the stance that they have some knowledge and expertise, which may be useful for the patient, but the patient is the ultimate author and director of their lives who can use the information as they see fit.

Summary of Ways to Respond to Resistance in CTNA

- Do not become defensive or justify the test results.
- "Roll with resistance" as is consistent with MI principles, where resistance is not met with confrontation but is understood from the patient's perspective.
- Acknowledge the strengths and weaknesses of neuropsychological tests.
- Be sure that the relationship between test results and the patient's daily functioning has been adequately illuminated.

Step 5: Summarizing the Relationship Between Tests Results, Life Areas, and Patient Questions

This is the part of the session where the clinician and patient work together to find the best way to use the test results to help make changes in important life areas and to answer questions the patient posed early on. This is highly individualized and depends a great deal on the direction in which the session has progressed. For example, some patients begin talking about the relationship between their cognition and life problems well into the session, so making the connection in the summary is merely a reminder. For others, they may be unable to see the connection until the clinician summarizes the different points discussed. This segment of the session is comprised of three areas, offering a grand summary, asking the patient how they would like to use the results, and answering questions and making recommendations.

1. The Grand Summary

In MI, the grand summary consists of the clinician providing a concise and relatively brief account of the major themes discussed in a session. This is the same for the CTNA feedback session; however, the grand summary can be more complicated because the clinician must summarize important points about cognition and personal themes the feedback has elicited from the patient. The CTNA feedback form contains a large quantity of information, and the discussion may cover many points. It may be helpful for the clinician to write down the main points as the session progresses. It is important to note that the grand summary does not require the clinician to simply regurgitate every little detail but instead to provide a concise summarization of the important themes that were discussed. A summary may be interactive and does not simply have to be a long dialogue by the clinician. Consider the following summary.

Clinician: I'd like to pull together everything we've been talking about, would that be ok with you?

Patient: Yes, sure. Good luck.

Clinician: It sounds like that as we've talked you are really seeing how this information applies to your life. Your strengths are that you're a good problem solver because you figure things out really well, you can think on your feet, and can really focus and pay attention when you need to and stay on the task at hand. What seems to get in your way of meeting your goals is that you do become distracted and feel lost at times, especially when you're stressed out, and this leads your mind to race and become disorganized so you forget things, lose track of where you're at, and ultimately your goals and plans fall apart. Does that sound about right so far?

Patient: I mean, it hits the nail on the head. I can't stay focused I end up all over the place, and the next thing you know, boom, relapse; I'm out using that drug again.

Clinician: And another thing we talked about is that this really seems to happen when you don't have any support or structure. It's like when you do have structure, it gives you the safety and security of something that it's hard to do in your mind, structure and organize yourself.

Patient: That's it, that's what I need to do, find that structure and keep it otherwise I'm gonna be right back were I started.

The above scenario demonstrates how a grand summary is used to provide concise information that the patient can use and think about. In this case, the patient was able to use the summary to develop their own ideas about how they can begin to use this information. The situation illustrated in this example is not uncommon with many drug-addicted patients. Many of them have trouble with executive functioning abilities of planning, organizing, and staying focused. When they are in structured environments, they tend to do well because the structure is provided for them. However, when they are on their own, they do not have the internal resources provided with intact executive abilities. As a result, they become lost, disorganized, and hopeless. Most of them think that the reason is that they are crazy, deficient, or have some other negative label. CTNA makes no judgments or labels but simply provides objective information about strengths and weaknesses, so patients can visually see what areas they need to improve. This approach seems to allow for greater internalization of these issues, which creates insight and hope that these problems can be solved.

2. Providing Information and Advice

The grand summary is the time in the session where the clinician may offer diagnostic impressions based on the test results. These results are highly individualized and depend on the test profile, clinical history, and impressions by the consulting psychologist.

Regardless of the association, the method for providing such information is the same and is conducted in an MI-consistent manner. The clinician first asks permission to provide the patient information that may be useful to them. Once the patient agrees, the second step is to provide the information in an objective nonjudgmental manner. In CTNA, it is important to provide the information in simple terms without using complicated jargon. It is also important to tell the patient that although the information is viable, it is not "set in stone," leaving the opening for other possibilities. Finally, it is important to elicit patient reactions after providing the information to process any feelings or reactions and maintain a collaborative relationship. The following scenarios provide examples of providing information. The first example is not consistent with MI.

Clinician: James after reviewing your profile, your cognitive impairments are likely due to your 20 years history of alcohol and 10 year history of using alcohol and cocaine together. Based on the research, individuals who use alcohol and cocaine together perform worse on various cognitive measures than those who use alcohol or cocaine separately. When taken together, alcohol and cocaine combine to form a compound called cocaethylene. Cocaethylene tends to impair dopamine transmission in the frontal areas of the brain, which is most likely the cause for your executive impairments. Abstinence would be the best measure for remediating these problems.

The problem with this summary is that it (1) is filled with too much jargon, (2) is too long, and (3) does not encourage an open dialogue, and (4) the spirit of the summary is more reflective of an authoritarian clinician imparting information to a passive patient.

The following is a more MI-consistent way to provide information in the same scenario.

Clinician: James we've talked about what the results of the tests mean for you. Would you be interested in hearing some thoughts I have about some of these results? [Closed-ended question asking permission to give information]

Patient: Yes, sure.

Clinician: I'm thinking that your cocaine and alcohol use may have contributed to some of the weaknesses we were looking at earlier. You mentioned that you have noticed a difference than before you started using drugs and it sounds like you saw yourself as pretty sharp, focused, and really "with it" in many different areas. [Providing information]

Patient: Yeah, I was really good at doing a lot of different things at once, it seems now I can barely complete one thing.

Clinician: Well there is information that cocaine and alcohol, especially when using it over a period of time, can really affect these skills that we've been talking about. Based on your history, there doesn't seem to be any other real good reason why your thinking would be this way so I have to assume that the cocaine and alcohol had the biggest effect. [Providing information in simple terms] What are your thoughts about that? [Open-ended question assessing patients' reactions to the information]

Patient: Yeah, it makes sense. I mean I've really noticed it about the last five years or so, that I really can't do things the way I used to. Does this get better?

This summary is more consistent with a collaborative approach because it (1) more openly enlists the patient's cooperation by asking permission, (2) is given in workable chunks versus a long drawn-out statement, (3) is stated in understandable terms, and (4) enlists the patient's thoughts and opinions about the information.

The above example shows how information provision is much more of a dialogue where the patient is an active collaborator versus a passive recipient. This is more effective in accepting the feedback, clarifying misconceptions, or modifying the information if so appropriate.

3. Using the Test Results

This is the next step in moving toward making recommendations. In CTNA, it is important to not jump right into making direct recommendations without first eliciting the patient's own ideas about how they would like to use this information. It is easy to fall into the expert trap and think that professional ideas or consultation will serve as an eye opener for patients. In reality, it places the patient in a passive and powerless recipient role without respecting that they may have ideas for how they want to use the information. Therefore, the first step would be to ask the patient how they would like to use the information and then use OARS to clarify their thoughts and perceptions. From there, the second step may be to gradually move into a change plan by specifying specific steps a patient will take to accomplish their goals. Consider the following example:

Clinician: So how can this information be used to help you, what have you gotten out of it and where do you want to go with it? [Open-ended questions]

Patient: The next step for me is that I have to learn to make decisions on my own.

Clinician: Ok, how are you going to do that? [Open-ended question]

Patient: I'm going to take my time, sit down and try not to let my thoughts go awry. I let my feelings override my thoughts and I get confused. It might sound crazy but that's what I need to do. I also need to find a balance between needing other people and standing on my own two feet.

Clinician: You need people but you also need independence. [Reflection of meaning]

Patient: Right, I need to be responsible. I have to sit back and analyze these things. I'm not lazy! Not at all! I want to be responsible and normal, whatever that is! That's what I learned here today, I want these things!

Clinician: The other thing is to focus, slow down and focus and use those problem solving skills that you have. [Simple reflection]

Patient: The focus is first. I've got to be focused.

The clinician can never be sure what information a patient will take as valuable to them, so it is important to roll with the patient's perception and not challenge it as invalid in some way. It would be easy, if what the patient learned is contrary to what the clinician thinks they should have learned, to fall into the trap where the clinician opinion is preeminent and that will likely shut the patient off from further dialogue. The best strategy is to elicit the patient's perception as to what they think they need to change, and then once that has been adequately addressed, offer information and recommendations as to what may be clinically helpful. Experience suggests that when patients' concerns are addressed in this manner, they are much more open to hearing clinician advice and suggestions and are more likely to consider them as viable options.

Patient: The thing is that I want this all right now! I want to feel better now! I know I can't think that way but I just get anxious. I think about everything that's happened and I don't want it to be that way, I want to fix it yesterday.

Clinician: When you think of all the consequences that have piled up from your accident it seems overwhelming and you'd like to make it just disappear. [Reflection of meaning]

Patient: Yes disappear, exactly, man I wish it could all just go away!

Clinician: And what happens when you think like that. [Open-ended question]

Patient: We'll I get really energized but somehow everything ends up going to hell and I end up saying to hell with it.

Clinician: And there were some things that came out of the test results that might be helpful in understand and working with this, would you be willing to hear them? [Providing information/closed-ended question asking permission to provide further information]

Patient: Oh yeah, yes.

Clinician: Remember we talked about what good problem solving skills you have but one thing that throws you off is when you don't have any structure? One thing I think that might help you is if you begin to think about what a structured rehabilitation program might look like for you and then take very small steps in working with that program. Saying that you have to keep all of your rehab meetings and do the recommended exercises is fine, but if you don't have a plan for meeting these goals, I'm thinking you'll become overwhelmed and frustrated again because you didn't think the whole process out. [Providing information]

Patient: That's usually what happens. I have good intentions and I really want to do this, but somehow I miss something from point A to point D or whatever.

Clinician: You don't think about points B or C. Or maybe even subpoint A1, A2, A3 [Reflection of meaning]

Patient: Or B1 or B2 (Joint laughter).

Clinician: Right, so what steps do you think you need to take in order to begin to meet some of these goals? [Open-ended question]

In this example, the clinician relates conflicts expressed by the patient to results from the neuropsychological tests. This creates a bridge of understanding between the assessment and the patient's real life. From that point, the clinician uses the test results as an avenue toward offering a suggestion for change. The patient is then more amenable toward hearing the clinician's ideas about change because (1) the clinician addressed the patient in an open and respectful manner, and (2) a bridge of understanding between the assessment results and the patient's real life was created.

This phase of the session is the beginning of a change plan, where the clinician and the patient work together to identify the steps to begin resolving life problems.

Summarizing the Relationship Between Test Results, Life Areas, and Patient Questions

- Provide a concise grand summary of the main points discussed in the feedback session. The grand summary is used to elicit thoughts from the patient regarding how they perceive the information and how they would like to use it to benefit their lives.

- Provide information and advice to the patient in an MI-consistent fashion.
- Use the test results to create a bridge between the assessment and the patient's real-world problems and concerns. This is done by first asking the patient how they would like to use the information and then providing any information and recommendations that are individually tailored to the patient's concerns.

Developing a Change Plan and Providing Recommendations

By the end of the grand summary, the patient and the clinician are likely to have some idea about what changes a patient wants to make. The stage is set to write down specific change plans and for the clinician to offer recommendations. These change plans can be written down on the last page of the CTNA feedback form. An important component of this phase is to encourage the development of a change plan but to watch out for traps that may hinder goal-setting efforts. Such traps include *underestimating ambivalence*, where the patient may still express uncertainty about goals they want to set or their commitment to implementing those goals. Evidence and experience suggests that patients who are pushed into change plans at the end of a session may actually show a decrease in their motivation to make changes (Amrhein, Miller, Yahne, Palmer, & Fulcher, 2003). Therefore, it is important to encourage but not push a change plan if the patient is not ready. In these cases, it is best to simply offer some recommendations while reinforcing that it is the patient's choice and responsibility to carry out the change plans. Two components of developing a change plan are eliciting ideas from the patient regarding what they would like to change and then providing recommendations in an MI-consistent manner.

1. Eliciting Patient Change Plans

The first step in developing a change plan is to elicit the patient's ideas about how they would like to use the information discussed in the feedback form. To initiate this conversation, the clinician begins with a "key question" (Miller & Rollnick, 1991, 2002). The key question is an open-ended question that asks the patient how they would like to use the information given and what kind of change plan they want to develop. The key question also provides valuable information to the clinician in regard to the patient's thought processes at this stage in the session and what kind of changes they are ready to make. Important knowledge to be gained from the patient following the key question includes the following: (a) what behaviors is the patient willing to change, (b) how ready are they to make these changes, and (c) what steps are they prepared to take that can be included in the change plan?

2. Behaviors for Change

The key question is designed to identify what behaviors a patient is ready to think about changing. Even if the CTNA session has progressed smoothly with little resistance, this does not necessarily mean a patient is ready for life-altering change plans. Therefore, it is important that the clinician relies on active listening skills and open-ended questions in order to clarify the patient's thoughts about change. Consider the following example with a patient who learned through the testing that she becomes highly anxious and dependent on others to make decisions for her: The result is that her anxiety causes her thoughts to race, she becomes unfocused and disorganized, and she is unable to make good decisions for herself.

Clinician: So how can we use this information to help you? What's the next step for you? [Open-ended key question]

Patient: The next step for me is that I have to learn to make decisions on my own.

Clinician: Ok, how are you going to do that? [Open-ended question]

Patient: I need to sit down and take my time and not let my thoughts go awry. I let my thoughts and feelings get the best of me and I get confused. Those are the kind of things that make me think of suicide. I know that sounds crazy....

Clinician: So you need to be able to contain your own thoughts so as to not rely on others so much to keep you together. [Amplified reflection]

Patient: Right, right.

Clinician: So finding a balance between including important people in your life yet standing on your own two feet when you need to. [Reflection of meaning]

Patient: Right and I think my depression is a big part of that. I want to find out more about what that's about. Because I didn't have this when I was really young it was when I hit my young adult years that I really noticed that and that's when everything started to fall apart.

Clinician: So it sounds like one thing you'd like to do is find out more about this depression you've experienced for a long time and gain some understanding about it and what might be causing it. [Reflective summary]

In this example, the scenario is that one part of the change plan was for the patient to receive more knowledge and education about depression, how it fits in their life, and what can be done about it.

3. Assessing Readiness

The next part of developing a change plan is to assess the patient's readiness to carry out the plan. This can be done by assessing the stage of change a patient is in regarding a particular behavior. One of the key insights developed through research on MI is that a patient's expression of a desire to change is not necessarily related to the likelihood that they will change. What does seem to be related to an increased likelihood of change is the *strength* of the patient's commitment to change. In MI, clinicians look for commitment language, which is reflected in the acronym DARN (desire, ability, reasons, need). However, commitment language itself has not been found to predict change.

It is rather the intensity of the commitment language that has predicted the likelihood of change in behavior (Amrhein et al., 2003). Therefore, it is important for the clinician conducting CTNA to listen closely to the intensity of a patient's commitment to a change plan. Otherwise, it may be erroneously assumed that a patient is ready for change when, in fact, this may not be the case. Consider the following scenarios.

Clinician: So, how would you like to use these test results to help your situation?
Patient: Well, I guess I should think about my long-term plans.
Clinician: So you're thinking about how to plan for your future?
Patient: Yeah, I suppose I am.
Clinician: Ok, are you open to some suggestions on how you might do this?
Patient: Sure.

In this scenario, although the clinician is not pushing or coercing the patient into a change plan, it is clear that the clinician has missed some underlying ambivalence that may be present. Words such as "I suppose" or "I guess" are more reflective of ambivalence and indecision than a true, solid commitment to change. Instead of glossing over the ambivalence and increasing the likelihood that the plan will not be followed, it would be advisable to address the ambivalence directly and develop a more realistic plan.

Clinician: How would you like to use these results to help your situation? [Open-ended question]
Patient: Well I guess I should think about my long-term plans.
Clinician: You're thinking it would be a good idea but you're not too sure? [Double-sided reflection illuminating ambivalence]
Patient: I mean...I don't know, I suppose I should.
Clinician: You seem uncertain [Simple reflection] Can you share your thoughts? [Closed-ended question]
Patient: I mean I know I need to think about a different future given my accident, and I know that these results are right, and I'm sure that my memory is pretty bad ... but I just don't know if it really makes that big of a difference.
Clinician: There are a lot of changes and it's hard to really know how things are going to be different now. [Reflection of meaning]
Patient: Right, how am I going to deal with things? I mean this is so different from the *me* I've lived with for 53 years.
Clinician: So the question is how you can adapt to the new you and plan for a realistic future for you and your family. It must be hard to think about that. [Reflection of meaning]
Patient: Yes, it just feels like giving up a little hope.
Clinician: Tell me about hope [Probing statement]

In this situation, the clinician identifies the ambivalence, reflects it back to the patient, and then offers a challenging question to encourage the patient to think of other possibilities. It would be easy for the clinician to say something like, "Yeah, but if you don't start making realistic plans, you and your family will face some bad times." Such a response uses the CTNA information almost as a threat. The clinician would essentially be trying to appeal to the patient's fear by saying, "If you don't change, then your family will suffer." This is *not* what the CTNA is intended to accomplish. The CTNA is not a fear tool. It is designed to provide objective information to the patient so that the patient can use that information in any way they see fit. The clinician acts as a guide to help the patient understand the information and what it means for their life. Certainly, there are situations where a clinician will tell a patient about possible consequences of their behavior. However, the clinician must not take the approach of using the information to scare or *make* the patient change. Instead, the clinician uses the information and the patient-centered style to *create an atmosphere where change is likely to occur.*

4. Providing Recommendations

The next step is to provide recommendations to the patient for treatment planning. These recommendations are highly individualized and are based on information acquired during the course of the feedback session and the results of the tests.

Recommendations are developed based on important themes elicited from the feedback session, information from the patient's cognitive profile, and life areas the patient is concerned about. The format for providing recommendations uses the framework "Elicit–Provide–Elicit." First, the clinician elicits ideas from the patient on what things they would like to put on a treatment plan; second, the clinician provides recommendations with permission; third, the clinician elicits patient reactions to the recommendations. Consider the following example of a patient who was concerned about their memory. In this situation, the patient's memory was actually quite strong, but she had problems with attention and working memory. Her attention and working memory problems were likely related to a history of drug use but also anxiety and depression she had been experiencing as a result of feeling overwhelmed in recovery.

Clinician:	Lori, have you given any thought as to how you would like to use this information we discussed today? [Eliciting patient ideas]
Patient:	Well, I'm relieved that my memory is ok, but I'm not sure what to do about my attention span.
Clinician:	Ok, well can I offer you some ideas? [Asking permission to provide information and recommendations]
Patient:	Yes please.

Clinician: I do think that your drug and alcohol use has affected some of the abilities we've talked about today. [Provides information based on clinical experience] However, I'm also struck by how overwhelmed you told me you've been feeling. You mentioned that raising your children, staying clean and generally trying to get your life together has been trying and at times you feel like you just want to sleep? [Summarizes what the patient said as a bridge to recommendations]

Patient: Yes that's right.

Clinician: Depression and anxiety can also affect some of the abilities we've been discussing [Providing information] What are your thoughts about that? [Elicits reactions to the information]

Patient: (Sighing in relief) I have been depressed and I've just been trying to ignore it. I just don't feel like I'm doing anything (beginning to cry). I mean I'm trying but I can't seem to get it together. Do you think my drug use has made me like this?

Clinician: Drug use certainly affects these things but you've been clean for a couple months, I think your depression and stress may be affecting this even more now. [Providing information] When you're depressed it's hard to focus and pay attention and it's easy to get overwhelmed. [Providing information] Does that fit for you? [Open-ended question]

Patient: Yes, very much so. I can't keep things straight in my head. A lot of it has to do with that I thought things would get better after getting clean but it seems to be getting harder.

Clinician: A lot of patients feel the same way. They get clean but then become overwhelmed with putting the pieces of their life together. Often they think their failing but really it's that their stressed, anxious, and depressed and that if they begin to address those things they begin to notice life smoothing out a bit. [Providing information based on personal clinical experience] Is that something you'd be interested in talking further about? [Open-ended question eliciting a commitment]

Patient: Yes definitely, I need to do something or I'm going to shut down.

Clinician: Are you open to some ideas from me? [Open-ended question]

Patient: Absolutely.

Clinician: Because you're already taking medication and that seems to be working for the most part, I would just encourage you to continue that. [Providing information]

Patient: Ok.

Clinician: The other part is therapy. What you might consider is focusing now on your daily tasks and routines and the way you feel. There are strategies called cognitive–behavioral strategies. They can help you learn self-management strategies. These are tools to help you organize and prioritize your daily routines in a way that seems workable and doesn't overwhelm you. In that way you're not just relying on your attention and memory to do these things, you have a concrete, visible plan for structuring your day that makes sense and doesn't leave you feeling overwhelmed and hopeless. [Providing information] Does that sound like something that would work for you? [Open-ended question eliciting patient thoughts]

Patient: Yes! That's what I need to do. I just try to figure things out in my head and it doesn't work. I have too much going on. How would this therapy work?

In this example, the clinician makes recommendations based on the test results, the patients' disclosures, and observations during the early parts of the session. Thus, the recommendations are tailor made for the patient and their needs versus being esoteric advice that may or may not fit the patient's life and needs. In addition, patient reactions to the clinician's observations and recommendations are elicited throughout the session. In this way, the clinician can make sure the recommendations fit the patient and that the observations are correct.

The main points for developing a change plan and providing recommendations are as follows:

- Ask a "key question" in order to elicit from the patient what changes they want to make.
- Assess the patient's readiness to make changes by assessing the stage of change and the strength of their commitment language.
- Provide recommendations based on themes from the feedback session, the patient's cognitive profile, and life areas the patient has expressed concern about.
- Provide recommendations using the format "Elicit–Provide–Elicit," always enlisting the patient as an active collaborator in the treatment plan recommendations.

Chapter 6
Putting It All Together: Two CTNA Case Examples

Case #1. Dementia or Pseudodementia?

This is a case of a woman we'll call Jane. Jane sought a neuropsychological evaluation from me (Dr. Gorske), after seeing a neurologist, initially for a second opinion regarding medical problems she was having, but in the process she revealed that she had been experiencing memory and concentration difficulties that were affecting her work. She told her neurologist that she had noticed memory difficulties for many years, but over the last year, these seemed to worsen. She was worried that she might have a serious neurological problem, such as dementia, so she wanted to be evaluated in order to either put her mind to rest or begin some type of preventative treatment. I received the referral from the neurologist, with a prescription indicating that the purpose of the evaluation was to assess for a dementia or a pseudodementia. Jane was scheduled for about 2 weeks later.

When I met Jane, her level of focus and sense of purpose struck me immediately. I met her in the waiting room, and she immediately stood up, shook my hand (firmly, I might add), handed me the initial demographic paperwork that was sent to her, and followed me back to my office. In her arm was a briefcase that I assumed was full of folders and paperwork. We did a little bit of small talk on the way back about her drive, the weather, among other things. However, it was clear that she was ready to get down to business.

During the initial history-gathering session, another thing that struck me about Jane was how informed she was about the purpose of our meeting. Many patients I see do not understand why they are there and have done no research about what to expect, and we usually spend time explaining what a neuropsychological assessment is, how it can be useful, and what can be expected from the results. Jane understood that this was a neuropsychological assessment to assess if she had a dementia disorder or a pseudodementia (which she did not completely understand, so I provided her information). She understood the basics of what was to happen and that it was a lengthy process. Afterward, I filled in a few other details about what she could expect. From there, she pulled out some of her paperwork and provided me with a list of doctors she wished to have the results sent to. Additionally, she provided me with a handwritten list of

T.T. Gorske, S.R. Smith, *Collaborative Therapeutic Neuropsychological Assessment*,
DOI: 10.1007/978-0-387-75426-0_6, © Springer Science+Business Media, LLC 2009

her medications and their side effects and a list of medical problems and procedures she had experienced in the last 15 years and the types of complications she experienced (cognitive or otherwise) as a result of these illnesses and procedures.

We proceeded to discuss relevant history. It is rare that I come across an individual who reports their personal history as detailed and succinctly as Jane. Jane was a Caucasian female in her mid-50s. She had a graduate degree and worked most of her life in administrative and management positions. By all accounts, she was a highly intelligent, competent, and insightful person who was a self-described "go-getter," who has historically been mentally sharp up until she began noticing her cognitive difficulties. Jane had a history of multiple medical problems, including fibromyalgia, irregular heartbeat, and hypertension (controlled at the time of our meeting), and she had a bout with cancer for which she received chemo- and radiation therapy. There was no evidence in her history of a head injury, seizures, loss of consciousness, or any other incident that could compromise her cognition. She had been experiencing bouts of depression for which she was on an antidepressant and received periodic psychotherapy, but her mood symptoms did not impair her functioning to any significant degree. She was, however, dealing with many stressful situations. Her one grown child had significant mental health issues leading to periodic hospitalizations. Jane was divorced, and her marriage had been conflictual and stressful due to her husband's severe mental health issues. These, in addition to her multiple medical issues, her chronic pain, and her fears of not being able to work, all weighed on Jane. Yet she relayed all these experiences in a calm, intelligent, and insightful way, admitting that the stress takes a toll on her but that she would never think of giving up trying to live a meaningful life.

Jane's family history included members with mental health and substance abuse problems, and there were at least two distant relatives that were suspected of having dementia. The knowledge of these family members is what made Jane nervous because she was afraid of following the same path.

After completing her history, we proceeded with the neuropsychological testing. Jane showed fine endurance and persistence and seemed to give her best effort throughout. Thus, I felt the results were likely a good estimation of her abilities. After completing the tests, we scheduled a feedback session for 2 weeks later.

Jane was anxious and excited about the feedback session. She found the neuropsychological tests intriguing (she had never been tested before), and she wanted to learn the results and how they fit into her life. Her two questions were whether or not there was evidence of dementia and, if not, what could be the reason she has trouble remembering names and events?

I decided to address her first question about dementia because this obviously weighed heavily on her mind and because, in her case, the answer was easy. Jane performed in the high-average to superior range on all tests of intelligence, auditory and visual immediate and delayed memory and recognition, attention and working memory, episodic list-learning memory, executive functions (with a few exceptions that will be discussed), and confrontation naming. All test scores fell between the 80th and 90th percentiles. Her memory was quite intact (and, in fact, probably better than mine!), and there were no signs of a dementing process based on her test results. This obviously put Jane at ease, but the question remained, why was she having these problems she's noticed?

We looked at her scores on the Controlled Oral Word Association Test (COWA), which included FAS and animal naming. Her scores on these tests fell in the average to low-average range, a considerable discrepancy, given her other scores. I asked Jane about her experience taking that test. She remembered that during the test, she began citing words that began with "F" and then had a brief moment of "blanking out." I asked her what was going through her mind at that moment. Jane looked at me and said that she was thinking to herself, "What is wrong with you? Are you stupid? You should be able to do this. You must be some kind of idiot?" I asked her what happened next. She stated that she began to become angry and berate herself for not being able to come up with more words. I then asked her if she noticed what happened to her when she was saying those things to herself. Jane thought for a moment and then began to nod and stated that she became more angry and tense, at which point her mind became a complete blank. I summarized the process Jane just described and asked her to tell me more about it.

Jane proceeded to tell me that she has always been very hard on herself. In work, with her children, and even when she was married to a severely mentally ill man, she placed high expectations on herself to take care of things and perform well. To perform meant to be a good mother, wife, worker, student, or whatever roles Jane adopted for herself. Whenever Jane felt she was not meeting expectations or, heaven forbid, actually failing at something, she would become very hard on herself and mentally berate herself. Usually this process was barely conscious to her. She recognized that she placed high demands on herself but had never fully realized the degree of harshness that was reflected in her thoughts. She recognized that she would become tense and unable to fluidly perform any task or duty, and she perceived herself as "shutting down."

Quite spontaneously, Jane then began to describe her early childhood years. She grew up in a family that expected high levels of achievement from her and her siblings. She further remembers never being able to please her parents for anything she did. If she brought home all *As* in school, there was no acknowledgement because that was to be expected. If she missed 1 out of 30 items on a test, she was asked why she missed that one. However, at the same time she received mixed messages. The boys in her family were held in high esteem, while the girls' accomplishments were overlooked. Jane never felt encouraged and validated in her competencies or accomplishments. However, instead of becoming hopeless, she tried even harder. The harder she tried, the more she achieved. However, the downside is that she became hypersensitive to any perceived failure. Any event perceived as a failure suddenly led her to experience a flood of anxiety while her past and present merged, and she began hearing a series of cognitive injunctions that she was incompetent and inadequate. The anxiety created from this experience led her mind to shut down from stress.

For the last 10 or 15 years, Jane had been trying to be a good mother, wife, employee, and student and concomitantly had been trying to effectively deal with her own failing health. I described her experience as trying to juggle all these competing demands, all the while feeling intensely anxious and incompetent until her mind finally says, "Enough, I'm taking a nap!" The experience of her mind taking a nap is that she does not process information quickly, efficiently, and fluidly. As a result, she does not attend to and forgets things. This process was best described in Jane's description of her feelings during the neuropsychological tests. Most people experience some level of anxiety during testing because of the inherent performance demands. However, Jane said she felt the most relaxed she'd been in a while because she only had to attend to one task for a period of time. Her exemplary scores reflected what she is capable of when she is able to focus and concentrate without being distracted by her multiple daily stressors and harsh internal dialogue.

Our conversation answered many questions for Jane. Hearing that she was extremely bright with an above-average memory capacity was very relieving and validating for her. Our discussion about the way she deals with stress was something she partially knew about herself, but she had no understanding of how it was impacting her. We discussed ways she could use this information in her psychotherapy meetings. I suggested that she learn ways to identify when this "stress reaction process" is occurring and then find ways to counteract her stress response through relaxation, meditation, and mindfulness training in addition to some traditional cognitive therapy work. I suggested that a mindfulness-based cognitive therapy intervention could be very helpful now that she is armed with this experiential knowledge of how her thoughts and beliefs about herself contribute to the stress response, which in turn leads to inefficient cognitive processing. In reviewing her history, I also suggested the possibility that her medical conditions, in particular her bout with cancer, chemo-, and radiation therapy could be contributing to some of her lowered cognitive abilities as well. However, I leaned more toward anxiety being the culprit and suggested that she work on these therapy strategies and undergo retesting in 1 year. Jane readily agreed to this and seemed anxious to begin working on these issues.

Comment: I have seen many cases like this where the patient is a highly intelligent and accomplished woman in her early to mid-50s, who gradually becomes aware of a decline in her cognitive abilities. Most of the time, the results are similar to those of Jane's. Occasionally, I have had the unfortunate experience where the cognitive decline fits a mild cognitive impairment profile, and further neurological examinations suggest the patient is in the very early stages of dementia or some other neurological condition. Other times, the reasons for the cognitive changes have been related to medical conditions and sometimes hormonal imbalances related to change of life. Yet other times, the change is perceived.

Patients compare their cognitive abilities to the way they were at age 20 instead of accepting that there is normal-age cognitive decline.

In the cases like Jane's, I am struck by the history of where the patient, usually a woman, has grown up in an environment that has been invalidating to their intellectual initiatives. Young girls receive the message(s) that their intellectual achievements are not important or that nothing they do is good enough. For me, such cases have driven home the importance of finding a balance between encouraging our young girls' achievements and competencies while accepting and validating who they are as human beings.

Case #2: Brian's Brain

Brian was a 9-year-old boy referred for an evaluation at the Psychology Assessment Center at U.C. Santa Barbara. After seeing an advertisement for our services, his mother brought Brian to our clinic for the evaluation of a possible attention-deficit disorder. He had a 2-year history of inattention in school, some minor behavioral disruptions, and deteriorating peer relationships. Approximately 9 months prior to his appointment, he was started on a stimulant medication by his pediatrician. According to Brian's mother, the medication had mixed effects; although it seemed to reduce the amount of outbursts in the classroom, Brian seemed lethargic and "directionless."

Brian's mother was a well-groomed professional woman in her late 30s. She and Brian's father, an architect, had been married for 12 years, and Brian was their only child. Both she and Brian's father had college degrees and worked fulltime in professional-level occupations. There was no family history of ADHD, learning disabilities, psychiatric disturbance, or significant medical problems. Pregnancy and delivery were unremarkable, and all developmental milestones were achieved on time or early. Brian's health history was likewise unremarkable. All reports stated that Brian was a healthy and happy child.

Apparently, trouble began midway through first grade, where Brian began to lose focus in the classroom. He was often off-task, and teachers frequently had to redirect him to maintain his seat, complete his work, and keep appropriate boundaries with other children. He continued to have friends and playmates, but as his behavior became increasingly disruptive, these friendships were more and more strained. His mother tearfully recalled Brian's dismay at not having been invited to a classmate's birthday party a year ago. His teachers strongly urged Brian's mother to seek a consultation for stimulant medication. She was initially resistant to the idea, and instead, took him for a nutritional analysis, hoping for a dietary change that might be helpful. After 3 months of a specialized diet, Brian's condition did not improve. Reluctantly, she discussed the issue with her pediatrician, and he was started on his first course of medication. After a discussion with his physician and his mother, it was agreed that he would not be tested while taking medication.

Brian eagerly presented for neuropsychological assessment. He was easily separated from his mother and accompanied the clinician to the testing room. Throughout the evaluation he was curious, engaged, funny, and delightful to work with. He easily persevered throughout the lengthy process and appropriately asked for breaks when necessary. Despite his relatively good mood, Brian would often make disparaging remarks about his own abilities. Comments such as, "Oh, I bet this will be hard," "I don't know if I can, but I'll try," and "I might have screwed that up, but I'm not sure" punctuated his test performance. When asked why he thought that his performance was poor, Brian would often shrug or say, "Because I'm not good at this sort of thing." The examiner pressed him further to describe other times that he feels like this. He responded, "I don't know. In school, a lot of the kids really seem to be able to get stuff quickly, but I'm not as smart as they are. I'm not quick like that." Later, he said, "I feel stupid compared to other kids." He was encouraged through the assessment to try his best, and he was praised frequently for his hard work and diligence. At the end of the evaluation, Brian's mother was sent home with behavior-rating scales for her, her husband, and Brian's teacher to complete and return via mail.

Results of behavior ratings did, indeed, suggest clinical levels of attention problems and hyperactivity, both at home and at school. His teacher noted higher levels of inattention, but his mother reported higher levels of hyperactivity at home. However, Brian's father's report did not acknowledge significant concerns for either hyperactivity or inattention, but rather reflected concerns about depression and anxiety.

Strikingly, Brian's test results are nearly uniformly strong. Measures of cognitive, achievement, and memory were all in the high-average to superior range, with little scatter. Given the reason for referral, Brian was administered several tests of executive functioning and attention. Results of the Rey–Osterrieth, Wisconsin Card Sort, a Continuous Performance Test, Stroop, and COWA revealed no difficulty with organization, planning, sequencing, working memory, or sustained attention. In short, Brian did not display the cognitive markers for ADHD.

Brian was also administered several tests of personality and emotional adjustment including the Personality Inventory for Youth (PIY), incomplete sentences, Roberts Apperception Test, and the Rorschach. Briefly put, consistent with his father's report, Brian appeared to struggle with issues of negative mood, poor self-esteem, and anxieties about personal abilities, safety, and expectations of others. Brian noted that he is often inattentive, but these concerns did not seem to be of the same magnitude as his affective issues. In short, the same indecisiveness and lack of confidence seen in Brian's test-taking behavior was noted in the results of his emotional assessment.

Four weeks later, Brian and his mother returned for feedback. Although Brian's father had initially hoped to be present, a last-minute meeting called him away unexpectedly. Because of Brian's age, it was decided to present testing feedback separately to him and his mother. The discussion started alone with his mother. Because the primary reason for referral related to the presence or absence of ADHD, this is where we began feedback. We began by asking Brian's mother how she expected that he did on the tests. "I don't know," she replied, "I'm assuming that he's pretty bright, but that he might've gotten really off track on things." To illustrate, we started by discussing the Continuous Performance Test that we administer via computer. After describing the nature of the test and that it was a good measure of sustained attention, she offered, "Oh boy, I bet he really bombed that." She was quite surprised to hear that he performed well on the task and all of the other measures of attention.

"So, what's going on?" she asked. Feedback went on to describe Brian's test-taking behavior, the comments he often made about himself, and his fears about the adequacy of his performance. "Does that sound like Brian?" we asked. She acknowledged that it did, but that she worried that this was a *reaction* to his cognitive problems. We went on to explain to Brian's mother that although he displays the behavioral symptoms of ADHD, these did not seem to have a primary cognitive origin. In our clinic, we call this a *functional ADHD*, meaning that the behavioral symptoms are present without any signs of cognitive correlates. In such cases, we begin to look for more social and emotional causes of inattention that might be attenuated by other forms of treatment, including psychotherapy, parent training, or family psychotherapy.

In attempting to answer the question of "the real issue," we spoke about the disagreement between her and her husband, which was reflected in the behavior-rating scales. "Well," she said, "Brian's father doesn't spend enough time with him to see all of these problems. He's often not around when trouble arises. When dad comes home, Brian is on his best behavior." We assured her that these scales did not communicate any *truth* about Brian's behavior, but rather were important in that they represented a disagreement about how they saw their son and the differential expectations they might have of him. We reflected, "How confusing it must be for Brian to have one parent who sees him like this [showing her dad's profile of scores] and one parent who sees him like this [showing her own ratings of Brian's behavior]. It can be difficult for kids to understand what's expected of them and whether they're a good kid or not." His mother responded, "Oh, I see what you mean. Things really haven't been very good at home between his father and me for some time now. We've been talking about separating and maybe even getting a divorce. Naturally, Brian doesn't know anything about this, but it's clear that we see him differently."

We went on to educate Brian's mother a bit about how children are often acutely aware of emotional issues between their parents, even if such issues are not discussed openly. We hypothesized that many, if not all, of Brian's symptoms might be explained by his fears about the integrity of his parents' marriage and his personal security in the midst of those issues. Brian's mother offered that maybe what was needed was some family psychotherapy to address these issues as well as some individual therapy to help Brian cope with the stressful situation.

Feedback with Brian was short, focusing mainly on reflecting to him that he was smart and that he should do well in school. The team acknowledged that we had "heard" Brian's emotional concerns and feelings that he often feels a little sad and worried about his abilities. We let him know that recommendations had been made to his parents about how they might be able to help him do as well as he possibly could.

In short, this case illustrates how testing data can reflect underlying issues that might not be neuropsychological at all. Brian's test-taking behavior was a great way to illustrate to him and to his mother that his issues were not cognitive ones, but emotional. Furthermore, rather than focusing on behavior ratings as a measure of Brian's *true* behavior, it was used to illustrate that there were different *perspectives* of him and what was causing his difficulties. These data can serve as a point of departure for future discussions, allowing all parties to begin with a common point of reference and a way of seeing their child.

Chapter 7
Applications of CTNA Methods

This chapter will discuss current and potential future applications of CTNA methods. Seven potential areas will be discussed, namely general clinical practice, rehabilitation, teaching, future research, cultural issues, children and adolescents, and the elderly.

General Clinical Practice

CTNA methods can be used in general clinical practice whenever neuropsychological assessment is warranted. The areas that CTNA methods are potentially effective include diagnostic clarification, treatment initiation, and development of treatment goals.

CTNA methods are well suited as a consultation method to provide diagnostic clarification for patients and their providers. Cognitive problems are common experiences with individuals who experience mild-to-severe emotional problems such as depression, anxiety, and others. For example, individuals with anxiety disorders often experience lapses in attention, concentration, and memory. Similarly, individuals with depression often have difficulty making decisions, paying attention, and remembering things. Even when the patient's mood or anxiety state has stabilized, there may be residual cognitive complaints that patients misinterpret as organic in nature. Depression and anxiety are often misinterpreted as symptoms of attention-deficit disorder or early Alzheimer's disease (AD). It is easy for patients to become confused about these disorders especially because of recent media attention to pharmacological therapies for adult attention-deficit disorder and early mild cognitive impairment as a precursor to AD. In conjunction with a detailed clinical history, CTNA methods can provide insight and clarification as to the nature of cognitive problems and diagnostic possibilities. Consider the following example:

A man in his early 50s diagnosed with bipolar I disorder and alcohol dependence had been able to maintain abstinence and a euthymic mood with the help of his treatment team. As time progressed, the man and his family noticed cognitive problems of forgetfulness, psychomotor slowing, inattentiveness, and a general

T.T. Gorske, S.R. Smith, *Collaborative Therapeutic Neuropsychological Assessment*,   105
DOI: 10.1007/978-0-387-75426-0_7, © Springer Science+Business Media, LLC 2009

lethargy that was not previously present. The man and his family began to worry that he had become "stupid" or brain damaged due to his years of alcohol use and psychiatric illness, and this created stress in the family and despondency in the patient. With the help of their clinician, they initiated neuropsychological testing. In the clinical history, there was no evidence of traumatic brain injury (TBI), stroke, or other major medical complaints. The test results showed the patient to be above average in general intelligence but in the impaired range on tests of information processing, attention, and concentration, which were affecting some of his immediate and delayed memory abilities. He also showed difficulty organizing his thoughts, which further contributed to his memory difficulties. His cognitive profile was most consistent with research and experience suggesting cognitive problems in euthymic patients with bipolar disorder. This information was given to the patient and the clinician in a team meeting. The feedback was reframed to the patient in the following way, "Sometimes with bipolar disorder, once the mood and behavior are under control, patients often notice their mind is out of control." This conceptualization made sense to the patient, and he and his family inquired about strategies for coping with cognitive problems.

In other situations, CTNA methods can be used to clarify methods and goals for treatment. For example, a young man suffering from a long history of psychiatric illness had maintained stability from mood symptoms for a significant period of time but was now experiencing anxiety that was creating functional problems. During the initial interview for anxiety treatment, the clinician began asking the patient open-ended questions designed to encourage the patient to elaborate on psychological conflicts. It became evident very early that these open-ended questions were making the patient highly anxious, and he began to "shut down" in the interview. On a hunch, the clinician asked the patient if he would be willing to take some brief neuropsychological tests, to which the patient agreed. The tests revealed that the patient had deficits in executive functioning, particularly working memory, mental flexibility, and abstract reasoning. It was clear that the patient had difficulty forming his own mental conceptualizations and became overwhelmed by his own thoughts, a symptom of his currently stabilized psychiatric condition. This likely explained reasons for his anxiety symptoms. The patient performed well in highly directive and structured situations, but became anxious and decompensated in less-structured and ambiguous situations. Therefore, an open-ended, nondirective type of therapy would be detrimental to the patient, so the clinician began a more structured and directive cognitive behavioral treatment. The patient became more relaxed and engaged and found the structured, written exercise of CBT to be very helpful in conceptualizing his own thought processes. The treatment was framed for the patient and his family as "teaching the patient to do on paper what he has difficulty doing in his mind."

As a final example, consider the case of a 25-year-old woman who was referred for a neuropsychological evaluation by her psychiatrist. This highly educated woman had a history of psychiatric hospitalizations secondary to depression and suicidal ideation. Despite her level of education, she was working as a custodian in a local hotel. She complained that her memory was poor, wondered if she had ADHD, and noted that she had made it through school due only to hard work and not to her intellect and that she was not generally cut out for a more complex or demanding occupation. Imagine her surprise when her WAIS-III scores revealed a full-scale IQ score of 146! Furthermore, scores on measures of executive functioning, attention, processing speed, memory, and organization were all similarly excellent. A comprehensive personality assessment also indicated that her mood issues were largely contained at the time of testing. The feedback focused on her continuing struggles with self-esteem, anxiety, and worries of decompensating into her prior psychiatric state. Bolstered by this feedback, she began to look for more intellectually satisfying work, considered graduate school, and even joined MENSA. In cases like this, the absence of neuropsychological findings can be as powerful and meaningful as a comprehensive picture of an evolving neurological condition.

These examples show how CTNA methods can be used in general clinical practice as either a consultation tool or a therapy initiator. Consequently, CTNA methods fit well into rehabilitation methods.

Rehabilitation Methods

Methods in rehabilitation of brain-injured patients date back to World War I, with the advent of improved neurosurgical techniques leading to increases in survival rates of head-injured servicemen (Boake, 1989). However, interest in TBI rehabilitation and research grew rapidly around 1979 coinciding with the foundation of the former National Head Injury Foundation, now the Brain Injury Association of America (BIAA) (Gordon et al., 2006). The proliferation of TBI rehabilitation research led to two comprehensive reviews. The first review concluded that there was a need for basic research in translating animal models to human clinical practice models, the need to better understand TBI recovery dynamics, the need for rehabilitation effectiveness evaluations and the factors affecting outcome, and the need to develop innovative service delivery models (NIH, 1999). A second review in 2005 provided evidence for cognitive rehabilitation's effectiveness with brain-injured patients such that the BIAA adopted a position paper in 2006, indicating that "Cognitive rehabilitation is central to the treatment and recovery of individuals with brain injury ...." (Katz, Ashley, O'Shanick, & Conners, 2006). One of the recommendations of the BIAA is as follows:

"Cognitive rehabilitation treatment strategies and goals, and the duration, scope, intensity, and internal of treatment should be determined based on appropriate diagnosis and prognosis, the individual functional needs of the person with brain injury and reasonable expectations of continued progress with treatment." (p. 15).

We believe that CTNA can be a valuable contribution to cognitive rehabilitation in the following areas: enhancing awareness of patients and their families of the need for cognitive rehabilitation and improving adherence to rehabilitation interventions.

Enhancing awareness. One challenge in cognitive rehabilitation is the ability to help patients recognize the need for an intervention in the first place. In this case, we are referring more to a psychological denial rather than a neurologically based lack of awareness such as anosognosia, although the two may be difficult to separate. Denial can be described as an emotional/subconscious process that interferes with intellectual awareness of a disability (Crosson et al., 1989). There is evidence that the level of acceptance or denial can have an impact on brain injury rehabilitation participation (Fleming & Strong, 1995; Katz et al., 2002; Schönberger, Humle, Zeeman, & Teasdale, 2006). CTNA's patient-centered and educational methods may be effective in providing patients and/or families in a way that does not lead to defensiveness and resistance and thus allows the patient to hear information that may be discrepant from their self-concept.

Improving adherence to treatment recommendations: CTNA methods are well suited for addressing treatment adherence issues. The person-centered style of administering CTNA serves to lower patient resistance and foster the development of a collaborative relationship. This, accompanied with objective, nonjudgmental feedback about cognitive strengths and weakness, and the effort to apply these skills to patient's daily life, may facilitate the development of insight and move the patient from a precontemplative state (no problem is perceived) to a contemplative state (the likelihood of a problem is considered). Pegg et al. (2005) illustrated the use of medical and neuropsychological information in TBI patients. Patients who received medical and neuropsychological information in a person-centered style of interaction experienced a sense of empowerment over their rehabilitative efforts and essentially became more informed and effective consumers of cognitive rehabilitation. In addition, CTNA methods fit well into Cognitive Rehabilitation Principles as cited in Prigatano (1999).

> Principle 1. The clinician must begin with patient's subjective or phenomenological experience to reduce frustrations and confusion in order to engage them in the rehabilitative process.
>
> Principle 4. Neuropsychological rehabilitation helps patients observe their behavior and thereby teaches them about the direct and indirect effects of brain injury.
>
> Principle 13. The rehabilitation of patients with higher cerebral deficits requires both scientific and phenomenological approaches. Both are necessary to maximize recovery and adaptation to the effects of brain injury.

CTNA can be incorporated as a treatment entry intervention to rehabilitation methods in order to facilitate a therapeutic alliance, provide objective and nonjudgmental information about cognitive strengths and weaknesses to patients and their families, and empower consumers to become active participants in the development of rehabilitative strategies.

Teaching

CTNA methods are teachable to students who wish to learn the "art and science" of neuropsychological assessment and thus become "human-science" practitioners. The two primary disciplines are psychological assessment methods and person-centered communication style.

Students should learn the basics of psychological testing and measurement of personality and cognition. This includes an understanding of relevant readings in psychological and neuropsychological assessment. Students should have exposure to intelligence and memory test batteries in addition to self-report and performance-based personality measures. The important skill to be learned is the applicability of individual assessments to real-world functioning. Students should know not only what cognitive or personality traits a test assesses but also how those traits operate in the real world. Therefore, students should be able to state cognitive and personality traits in real-world terms that apply to daily life and functioning.

There is no standard way for teaching students a person-centered style of interacting with patients. Such instruction is generally left to the individual teacher based on his or her own knowledge and competence (see Handler & Hilsenroth, 1998 for an excellent review). Miller and Rollnick (1991, 2002) have developed and explained person-centered methods in a concrete and teachable format with Motivational Interviewing (MI). They illustrated the process of an MI session, provided an explicit method for giving feedback in a person-centered style, and developed adherence scales for assessing clinician competence in using MI skills. Thus, MI methods can be effective in teaching students to be person-centered practitioners. In addition, MI followers have written extensively on different training methods (see MI website, www.motivationalinterview.org).

Future Research

CTNA methods were originally developed with mentally ill substance abusers (MISA) patients. However, CTNA methods can generalize to a wide range of patients in many different settings. The study at the University of Pittsburgh School of Medicine in Addiction Medicine services examined the effects of the CTNA on patients diagnosed with substance dependence and a depressive disorder. This study examined the effectiveness of the CTNA in enhancing adherence rates, with patients entering an intensive partial hospital treatment program. The main outcome was the number of group sessions patients attend compared to the number of sessions they are required to attend. In addition, we examined patients' responses to the CTNA on a case-by-case basis to assess responsiveness to, and satisfaction with, CTNA. It is hoped that this information will help in the continual development and refinement of the intervention in order to optimize its usefulness and effectiveness.

Future studies can examine CTNA's effectiveness on these and other variables with different populations. For example, one area of recent interest has been the development of interventions for families of patients diagnosed with AD. Recent studies have shown that family mental health and functioning can have an impact on the quality of care patients with AD receive. It would be interesting to examine if the provision of objective and understandable cognitive feedback presented in a person-centered manner can have an impact on family members' understanding of the disorder, facilitate insight and understanding of the patient's functional strengths and weaknesses, and provide direction and hope as to what kind of interventions and resources are available to help families cope with the progressive decline of the disease.

Current research underway at the University of Santa Barbara by Dr. Steven Smith examines the use of neuropsychological test feedback to children and their families. For children diagnosed with attention-deficit disorder, learning disabilities, or other problems compromising cognitive ability, objective and nonjudgmental feedback may facilitate insight and understanding on the part of the patient and family members and provide direction for treatment.

Recent research has examined the effects of cognitive rehabilitation on patients diagnosed with a severe mental illness such as schizophrenia or bipolar disorder. Studies have reported the effects of cognitive deficits in hindering treatment planning and implementation. Future research can examine the use of CTNA methods as a consult to patients, families, and providers to provide insight and direction for more applicable treatment planning that considers patient's functional abilities. Thus, cognitive remediation can be more focused, and the patient can feel empowered as an active collaborator of the treatment process.

These are just some examples of areas where CTNA methods can be used in clinical practice, teaching, and research. It is our hope that professionals will consider adopting CTNA methods for the benefit of their patients. We also hope that instructors of psychological and neuropsychological testing will consider adopting these methods for their students. In doing so, we hope to disseminate a more collaborative and person-centered neuropsychological assessment process that enlists patients as partners in enhancing their health and well-being and empowers them to take charge of health decisions. Dr. Ronald Ruff has called for neuropsychologists to become "caretakers of cognitive health." We would expand upon that and call upon neuropsychologists to empower patients to become caretakers of their *own* cognitive health. We believe CTNA methods are a potentially powerful tool in the fulfillment of this goal.

CTNA and Cultural Issues

The field of neuropsychology has made strides in developing more culturally sensitive neuropsychological assessment and interpretation methods; however, there remains much to be done (see Fletcher-Janzen, Strickland, &

Reynolds, 2000, Handbook of Cross Cultural Neuropsychology for an excellent resource). The challenge is to develop a perspective in clinical neuropsychology that emphasizes understanding an individual's behavior in the larger context of their social milieu. This requires an understanding of brain–behavior relationships (and how they may have changed, given a specific experience, change, trauma, or other event), in the context of an individual's culture.

The strides that have been made in developing a culturally sensitive neuropsychology include norm-based scoring that integrates the influence of different ethnic groups, the literature on the impact of culture on cognition, and a general increased sensitivity by practitioners, teachers, and researchers as to the influence of social and contextual factors on brain–behavior relationships. Despite these strides, different ethnic groups continue to be suspicious of the assessment and testing process due to concerns of over-pathologizing, misinterpretation of symptoms, inaccurate attributions of symptom presentation and behavior, and misdiagnosis (Fletcher-Janzen et al., 2000). Such concerns often lead to poor clinician–patient rapport and a general environment that is unsupportive, defensive, and potentially hostile. Such an environment is easily created when a practitioner follows an information-gathering model of assessment where information is hidden from patients. Culturally diverse patients, who already feel suspicious of health care, testing, and assessment, are likely to become increasingly suspicious when an "alien" neuropsychological procedure is administered with little or no input from the patient.

CTNA methods are well suited for creating a more open, supportive, and culturally sensitive environment for the following reasons.

CNTA methods emphasize an open sharing of results. As opposed to the information-gathering model, where the emphasis is on *secrecy*, CTNA emphasizes *transparency* on the part of the clinician. This openness can reduce patient's feeling that there is a hidden agenda on the part of the professional. Many individuals from different cultural groups have knowledge and experience that professionals use tests to harm versus to help. CTNA makes the agenda of the assessment and feedback clear and open. In this way, the patient understands fully what is happening and what interventions or plans may arise from the testing and assessment process. An important part of this process is an open sharing and explanation of norm-based scoring and the strengths and weaknesses of neuropsychological tests. CTNA methods emphasize an open discussion about the strengths and weaknesses of norm-based scoring and how data may or may not apply to an individual's experience. This leads to the second reason why CTNA methods help create a culturally sensitive environment.

CTNA emphasizes the patient's perception of how their performance applies to their daily life. In CTNA, the clinician does not provide information in a "top-down" manner, where a patient passively receives knowledge from the clinician. CTNA emphasizes a two-way dialogue, reflected in the "Elicit–Provide–Elicit" method where clinicians seek to understand the meaning of knowledge and data for a patient. Such a dialogue could potentially segue into a conversation about social and cultural issues. Consider the following example with an African-American male patient in his early 40s, who dropped out of school in the 10th grade.

Clinician: Ok, Robert, this next is called the "Block Design" test. This is the test where I gave you a bunch of blocks with some sides red and some sides white and asked you to make patterns with them. Do you remember that test?

Patient: Oh yeah, I remember that test. It was frustrating as hell (laughs).

Clinician: Ok, can you tell me more about that?

Patient: Yeah, I mean the first ones were ok, but as it went on I couldn't figure out what was going on. I've never been interested in puzzles so I didn't think I'd do all that well.

Clinician: It sounds like as soon as *you saw what the test was about* you didn't think you were going to do very well.

Patient: Yeah, no way. Nothing I did seemed to fit. How did I do?

Clinician: Well, if you look at this graph here, you can see that your score fell in the 15th percentile. We would say that score falls in the low average range.

Patient: So that means I'm dumb, right?

Clinician: No, it means you fell in the low average range for *this* test. What I'd like to know is what did you see yourself having to do to work on this test?

Patient: (Thinking). I mean I had to guess the patterns, right? I had to figure out what goes where, like putting a puzzle together.

Clinician: Right, it's very much like putting a puzzle together. For this test you have to be able to look at the design, figure out the pattern in your mind, and then look at the blocks and piece them together in the right way. People who are good at this test are usually good at figuring out patterns to things, like an engineer. They can look at different parts of something and then put them together to make a whole picture.

Patient: (Nodding) Ok, yeah, we'll that's something I've never been good at. I mean, in school I remember trying to do puzzles, or things my teacher wanted me to do with my hands, and I just never got it. A lot of my friends were pretty good at mechanics and stuff like that but none of it made any sense to me.

Clinician: So this is something you've seen in yourself for a long time?

Patient: Yeah, so let me ask you something. What is this test about for black people and white people? I mean like...if a white person did the same way on this test, what would that mean as opposed to me doing how I did?

Clinician: Just so I'm clear. Are you asking if I would interpret this differently for you versus a white person?

Patient: Yeah, yeah that's it.

Clinician: That's a real good question. In my experience there are a couple different ways of thinking about it. In the past, some people have thought that blacks are not as smart as whites so that's why they don't do as well. But now we know that a lot of it boils down to opportunities. Whites tend to have more opportunities than blacks do and so they have better educational experiences and then do better on these types of tests. But I guess I'm wondering what you think about that and what you think is right?

Patient: (Leaning forward, showing greater interest) Man, I wanted to do good in school early on. In fact I was really good at things like poems, art, drawing and stuff like that. But where I come from, you get into that stuff and people think you're a punk and that doesn't help you on the street one bit. I mean, my dad was never around and my aunt raised me because my mom was usually doing her thing. My cousins would tell me that my education was out there not in school.

Clinician: So early on you really wanted to learn these things but it just wasn't supported where you came from because you needed to survive?

Patient: Yeah man, I know I'm not stupid. No offense but you'd get cut where I come from and I flow through it like water. (Clinician and patient laugh)

Clinician: I have no doubt, but can we talk some more about this? (Patient nods in agreement).

This is an example of how CTNA methods can create an open dialogue that explores the meaning of a test score for a patient without prematurely diagnosing and labeling them. In addition, the method emphasizes egalitarianism, where the clinician and patient are on equal footing. Here the patient can tell the clinician what the score means, instead of the clinician dictating to the patient. In this way, CTNA methods can create a bridge of understanding between cultures.

CTNA with Children, Adolescents, and Families

Clinical experience suggests that one of the challenges in helping family members whose child has been cognitively compromised, due to either injury or illness, is to be able to provide help and resources to the family while maintaining a positive working alliance. When a family has a child who has been injured, is not developing normally, or is behaving in some aberrant manner, the family looks to professionals for help and support, yet there is an air of suspicion at the same time. Families are very sensitive to feeling blamed, ashamed, and generally feeling as if their child's difficulties are their fault in some way, in addition to the helplessness they feel in regard to their inability to help their child. What they don't need is to be made to feel blamed and talked down to in a way that further disempowers them and lowers their motivation in wanting to accept help from professionals. Consider the following example of a family who has been struggling with their son's behavior problems and was referred for a neuropsychological evaluation by their pediatrician.

Clinician:	Good afternoon Mr. and Mrs. Jones, I'm going to give you some feedback about how Jimmy did on the tests he took, are you ready to hear all this?
Mr. Jones:	(After looking at Mrs. Jones, who is nervous and wringing her hands). Yes, I suppose so; can you tell us exactly what kind of information we'll be learning here?
Clinician:	Of course. We're going to help Jimmy. We're going to get him on the right track so that things can be better for all of you. (Mr. and Mrs. Jones smile slightly, but still appear worried).
Clinician:	Ok, so let's proceed. Basically Jimmy falls in the category of attention deficit disorder, predominantly hyperactive type. He displays the type of dis-inhibited behavior in addition to various executive, sequencing, and discrete attention abnormalities that I would expect in a child with such problems. His behavior during testing was quite poor. He displayed various impulsive and off tasks behaviors that made the session significantly longer than normally expected. Thus, I can see why the schools are having such problems with him. I would suggest immediately having him evaluated for medication and begin some mobile therapy and therapeutic staff support services.
Mrs. Jones:	(Beginning to cry but looking confused). Wait, how did you come up with all that? You can tell all that from the tests?
Mr. Jones:	(Irritated). What exactly did he do that tells you this? I can understand him being impulsive and off task, but you said "executive" what does that mean?
Clinician:	Really that's all semantics. The point being that his profile is very consistent with the diagnosis and I want to discuss recommendations. Now what we know is . . . . . .
Mr. Jones:	(Interrupting). Wait a minute! You're telling us he has this disorder! I've read about this. Don't these kids basically become screwed up, using drugs, killing their parents and things like that?
Mrs. Jones:	(Crying). No, I've heard they grow out of it. He'll grow out of it right? (Mr. and Mrs. Jones start talking back and forth).
Clinician:	I'm really rather taking aback that the two of you would be surprised by this. The rating scales you filled out were clearly significantly above the normal range so you must have had an indication that something was going on. Mr. Jones, didn't you tell the interviewer that you had some hyperactivity growing up? ADHD has a high level of genetic transmission so. . . . .
Mr. Jones:	So this is my fault he's this way? I have an M.B.A and a successful business, how can you compare me to Jimmy?

Clinician: Look, there are many good educational resources for you. There's an organization called CHADD that can help you understand this better. I think you just need some time to let this sink in. (Mr. and Mrs. Jones look at the table, despondent).

This interaction reflects a traditional information-gathering type of feedback model. The clinician talks to the family in an authoritative, top-down manner that leaves the family confused and disempowered and increases their resistance. CTNA methods enlist the family as an important source of information for understanding what a child may be going through. Consider an alternative way in which part of this interaction might progress.

Clinician: Mr. and Mrs. Jones, I'd like to share some observations with you about Jimmy in regards to how he did on the test and also some behaviors I saw, does that sound ok to you.

Mrs. Jones: Yes absolutely.

Clinician: Great. In regards to his test performance, one thing I saw was that Jimmy had a real hard time with tests that measure skills of attention and working memory. By attention, I mean that he just did not seem to be able to focus for any length of time, maybe a minute or two at most. Working memory is basically the ability to hold ideas in his mind and do something with the information. For example when I read him a series of numbers and letters that he had to put in the right order, he became frustrated and irritated very quickly. In fact he became irritated on many tests which would lead him to start moving around, getting out of his seat, acting rather silly, and inappropriately playing with the test materials. I'm wondering if any of this sounds familiar to you?

Mrs. Jones: (Both Mr. and Mrs. Jones are nodding). Oh god yes! When I try to talk to him, he's all over the place. I tell him a few simple things I want him to do and then he just looks at me and goes "huh". I mean, our daughter does that once in awhile, but for him it's constant. I can't keep him in one place.

Mr. Jones: Or keep him focused. I tried to take him fishing one time, I figured maybe I wasn't spending enough time with him and that might help. I tried to show him some simple things about baiting a hook. Dammit, he was all over the place! He couldn't listen even for a second! Finally, I thought, well maybe he just needs to try it himself. Well, stupid me! That's how he got that hook in his finger! I tried to hold his hand to get it out, because it wasn't that deep. But he kept fighting me, screaming, and flailing around that he hit his hand on the ground and shoved the hook deeper. Fortunately Children's Hospital wasn't too far away, but the drive there was hell.

Clinician: Wow! Obviously, we're seeing similar things. Also, I hear how frustrating it's been and it also sounds like you've been really wracking your brains trying to help him but nothing seems to work.

Mrs. Jones: Oh, god I feel horrible more than half the time (crying). Do you have any idea what's going on?

Clinician: Everything that I'm seeing on the tests and in the descriptions of Jimmy's behavior from you and the school seems to be consistent with Attention Deficit Disorder. Do you understand what that is and what it means?

Mr. Jones: I've read some things. What is it you're seeing that tells you that?

Clinician: Based on the markers we use, inability to pay attention, acting impulsively, unable to organize himself like at school and home (family nods), and the fact that this happens in many different areas of his life, are all consistent with this diagnosis, especially given that there appears to be no other real good explanation for any of these things. How do the two of you feel about what I'm saying?

Mr. Jones: I mean, everything your saying sounds right. You've captured Jimmy pretty well. But what can we do about this?

Clinician: Yes, let's move to that. What I'd like to do is talk to you about a number of options for helping Jimmy. The important thing is that we find a plan that fits for the both of you and that Jimmy can work with. How does that sound? (Both Mr. and Mrs. Jones nodding)

In this scenario, the clinician takes time to attend to the families' feelings, talks to them in a collaborative way using down-to-earth language instead of jargon, and emphasizes the importance of an individualized care plan that considers their needs and the needs of their child. Such an approach potentially empowers a family and motivates them to want to work with the clinician and find different ameliorative strategies.

The importance of CTNA as a tool to empower families cannot be understated. In dealing with schools, organizations, hospitals, and other systems, families often feel disempowered, overwhelmed, and at the mercy of the more knowledgeable and powerful system advocates. CTNA arms families with knowledge and skills in order to face such challenges and become an advocate for their child. Families can then feel like informed and empowered consumers of health-care knowledge that allows them to take charge of their own and their child's health and well-being.

CTNA with Elderly Patients and Their Families

Although there are many reasons elderly patients may be referred for a neuro-psychological assessment, most are referred for being assessed for a diagnosis of dementia or a mood disorder (Brown & Wiggins, 2005). This is consistent with my own (Dr. Gorske's) observations in clinical practice. The majority of patients I see are referred to determine a depression versus dementia diagnosis, to assess the aftereffects of a stroke, or to provide differential diagnosis of vascular cognitive impairment or a progressive dementia disorder. With patients whose cognition has not been severely compromised to the degree where comprehension, insight, and ability to process verbal information are impaired, I find the provision of feedback to be helpful to them and particularly to their loved ones. The patient-centered and collaborative feedback process appears to be helpful in ways already discussed throughout his book. The question remains, what role does a collaborative feedback method have for patients who have been severely cognitively compromised due to dementia, a severe mood disorder, or other neurological conditions where individual feedback is not appropriate and family involvement is essential? We believe that the importance of CTNA for family members of elderly patients lies in the ability to maintain a strong collaborative, working alliance that enlists family members as treatment team members and lowers their resistance to hearing difficult and possibly discrepant information.

Neuropsychologists are in a unique position to provide comprehensive and competent services to family members of patients who have been cognitively compromised. The challenge is for the clinician to broaden their clinical role as one who is knowledgeable in brain–behavior relationships and to understand the needs of family systems. With elderly patients, an event such as a diagnosis of dementia or depression creates imbalance in family systems to a point where longstanding family roles have now been shaken. The family homeostatic system has changed because the previously held role by the *patient* has now changed due to the event leading to cognitive difficulties. Family members therefore present to professionals with a myriad of assumptions, concerns, and emotional reactions that have the potential to influence the course of treatment planning and interventions (for reviews of these issues, see Storandt & VandenBos, 2005).

As a result of these issues, the neuropsychologists' clinical skills are of primary importance in providing feedback to elderly patients and their families for two reasons: the need to maintain a positive and collaborative relationship with family members and when providing feedback regarding the outcome of the evaluation. Maintaining a positive rapport with the family is essential in order to create an atmosphere of collaboration and empowerment that enlists family members as active treatment team members. As previously stated in this book, such an atmosphere is more likely to lead to successful development, implementation, and follow through with treatment recommendations.

The second issue, providing outcome information, refers to the often difficult situations neuropsychologists find themselves when providing test feedback information. A neuropsychologist may find themselves being bearers of bad news, which requires them to take the role of a supportive psychotherapist who tends to family members' thoughts and feelings about the information provided. In addition, this requires an understanding of family system's issues and dynamics. Another part of providing outcome information is the fact that neuropsychological assessment information may not provide definitive information about diagnosis or reasons for cognitive changes in a family member. This places the neuropsychologist in an awkward position to justify and clarify the strengths and weaknesses of neuropsychological assessment information (for an excellent in-depth review of these issues, see *Neuropsychological Evaluation of the Older Adult: A Clinician's Guidebook*, by Joanne Green).

CTNA methods are well suited for helping neuropsychologists with these issues identified above. CTNA provides a framework for interacting with family members in a collaborative way that addresses and deals with their emotions and potential resistance. Additionally, CTNA offers a framework for discussing the strengths and limits of neuropsychological assessment information yet emphasizes its importance in describing patient's cognitive and behavioral functioning. Consider the following example.

An 87-year-old woman is hospitalized for severe depression. She has had bouts of depression in the past (the last being over 20 years ago) and was tried on various medications and ultimately received electroconvulsive therapy (ECT), which appeared to have modestly positive effects. In order to assess her ability to receive ECT again, she undergoes numerous medical evaluations in addition to a neuropsychological consult to rule out any evidence of a more severe cognitive problem. The neuropsychologist and other treatment team members meet with the family and the patient to discuss the results. There are three family members present: the patient's oldest son and his wife and the patient's youngest daughter (all adults in their late 50s). The results of the neuropsychological examination are most consistent with a major mood disorder, and there is no evidence of a dementia process.

Clinician: Welcome to everyone. I'm glad you all were able to make this meeting. What I wanted to do was discuss the results of the neuropsychological evaluation your mother took so we can move on with her treatment. How does that sound to everyone?

Daughter: Ok wait. I'd like to know why she had to do this. They've been poking and prodding her all week and nobody seems to be doing anything. All that seems to happen is test after test but nothing else, so I'd like for you to explain what you're testing and what good is going to come of it.

Son: Maybe if you'd give the man a chance he might (Son and daughter stare at each other).

Wife: Ok let's let the doctor explain. Go ahead doctor.

Clinician: Ok, well basically your mother is not demented. She is actually pretty sharp mentally. So really I think we can talk about beginning....

Daughter: Sharp mentally? Have you been observing her? Does she look "sharp mentally" to you? (Points at the patient who is slouched in her chair, looking at the floor, silent)

Clinician: Ok what I'm trying to say is that while she is certainly very depressed, there is no evidence of more severe cognitive problems that would keep her from beginning ECT treatment.

Son: Ok but doctor, with all due respect, she is not "with it". This is a woman who was seeing things only two weeks ago and couldn't remember the names of my children. So I'm a little confused by you saying that she doesn't have severe cognitive problems. (The patient looks up as if wanting to say something)

Clinician: (Maintains eye contact with the son to other family members exclusion) But there are many things that can explain that. So far all tests indicate that she does not have dementia. What I'm trying to say is that. . . . .

Daughter: Then what does she have? I'm tired of people saying what she doesn't have and explaining the water! So why can't she lick this. Why are we here again? Mom, what's going on with you?! You've been doing this for over 30 years!

Patient: (After a pause and shrugging her shoulders) I don't know.

This brief example illustrates some of the challenges in providing information to family members. The goal of feedback in regard to elderly patients and their families is to provide information about diagnosis and education about a disorder and possible interventions. The difficulty here is the family context influencing the nature of the feedback session (Knight, 2005). The family context refers to the history, dynamics, and emotions family members bring into a feedback session. If these are not addressed and processed, there is the risk of increased resistance by family members, which leads to a breakdown in communication and collaboration. The clinician may be forced to "take over the session" or withdraw. Taking over the session may lead family members to feel disempowered and lead to passive resistance. Withdrawing may lead to the family members completely taking over the feedback session, and no useful knowledge is disseminated or gained.

CTNA methods challenge the clinician to play two primary roles. In the first role, the clinician is a knowledgeable neuropsychologist who is an expert in brain–behavior relationships and the meaning of those relationships to a person's life and functioning. The second role is one of collaborator and, in this case, an empathic group manager. The clinician uses the person-centered methods of CTNA to create an open yet structured therapeutic milieu that respects each person's perceptions and opinions, and uses that information for the benefit of the patient and the family in developing intervention strategies. Here's how the above scenario might look in such an atmosphere.

Clinician:	[Provides family members a copy of the neuropsychological test results] Good afternoon everyone. I want to thank all of you for coming here today. My name is Dr. John Smith. I'm the neuropsychologist in this treatment setting. I would like to ask if everyone knows what this meeting is for and what we're going to accomplish? [Introductory statement assessing family members' understanding of the meeting]
Son:	Well, to help mom I figured.
Daughter:	No clue.
Clinician:	Ok, Nancy (the patient), how about you? Do you know why we're meeting? [Assessing patient's comprehension of the meeting's purpose]
Patient:	Well, I guess it's about all those tests I took with you?
Clinician:	That's right. (Addressing family members) I'm a neuropsychologist. What that means is that I test different mental skills people have, like the ability to pay attention, remember things, solve problems, and other types of skills. I test people to assess how strong or weak they are in these areas and can often answer different questions based on the results. [Provides a framework for the session by describing neuropsychological assessment tasks]
Son:	Like what kind of questions?
Clinician:	Well, in this case, I've been asked to assess if there are any severe cognitive problems that might keep her from undergoing ECT treatments. So what I would like to do is tell you what I've found. How does that sound to everyone. [Provides a specific focus for the session and assesses family perceptions with an open-ended question]
Daughter:	So I want to know why she's having these episodes again after all these years. Can you tell me that?
Clinician:	That's a really good question, but I want to be clear and up front that I wasn't asked to determine that, nor do I believe that I could at this time. So no, I'm afraid I won't be able to answer that. Do you think that will affect how you see our work today? [Affirms family members' need for information; provides direct information and then assesses family members' readiness to proceed]
Daughter	(Sighing). Then it's just another damn meeting! When are these going to end? Nobody can seem to answer that!
Clinician:	(Attending to the daughter but then to the entire family) I hear this has been a long road for everyone and that it's been frustrating not to receive the answers you're looking for. [Reflective response]
Son:	Yes it has. While I don't agree with Terry (the daughter) that this is waste of time, it is hard not feeling like any progress has been made.
Daughter:	I didn't say it was a waste of time, don't put words in my mouth! I've been the one taking care of her when things get bad, so I have a right to know what's going on!

Clinician:	It's been hard on you, Terry, feeling like you've had to do a lot yourself with little support [Reflective statement] (Terry starts to tear up; clinician addresses the patient) Nancy, what are your hopes for our meeting today? [Enlisting the patient as an important session contributor]
Patient:	I want to get better. Will this help me get better?
Clinician:	What it will do, is tell us whether you are a good candidate for a treatment we hope will help you get better. How does that sound to you? [Provides information; elicits patient response]
Patient:	Ok, I'm ready.
Clinician:	For these tests what I look for are markers suggesting a severe problem with Nancy's mental skills. What I found is that she scored low on tests I would expect for someone with severe depression. However she scored well in the average range on tests that might suggest more serious cognitive problems. For example, her score on this test called Digit Symbol was quite low because she performed slowly. People with depression often perform very slowly on different tests. However, on a test of memory, where she had to remember a list of words, she actually did quite well for her age. So what that suggests is that she can remember information, she just isn't very fast taking it all in. How does that fit for what others are seeing? [Provides information in layman's terms; elicits family reactions]
Son:	So her memory is ok but she isn't very quick?
Clinician:	Yes, that's a good way of putting it. [Affirms family members' efforts to understand]
Son:	(Looking at his wife) Yeah, I can see where that fits. Sometimes she seems really forgetful, but other times she remembers stuff I'm surprised she remembers.
Clinician:	Can you give an example? [Elicits further information]
Wife:	I know one. About two weeks before she had that really bad episode, she was able to tell my brother every detail about our children's activities that I told her over the phone just a few days prior. But when she was in the midst of her episode, she didn't remember that I'd brought her some casserole earlier in the day.
Clinician:	So when she's feeling ok, she seems to remember things pretty well. But when she's depressed, her memory is worse. [Summarizes what the family members said in a concise manner]
Daughter:	So that means she's not demented?
Clinician:	What has been described is more consistent with severe depression than dementia. When an older person is more depressed, they can often look like they're demented but in fact that's not the case. Nancy, what do you think about what we're saying? [Provides information; elicits patient reaction]
Patient:	Oh, I know what's going on a lot better than you all think I do.

In this brief example, the clinician did a number of things consistent with CTNA methods. First, the clinician established a supportive, collaborative, yet focused framework for the session by describing the purpose while ensuring that family members understand the goals so that any inaccurate assumptions can be addressed early. Second, the clinician reflects and empathizes with family members' perceptions, particularly the family member who was most distressed. Feeling heard and understood, the family member may be more amenable to information that is hard to hear. Third, the clinician frequently summarizes what has been said so that there is no misunderstanding and elicits the family members' reactions to the summary. Fourth, the clinician attends to all members of the family instead of focusing on just one. This way, all family members feel a part of the process. Finally, the clinician enlists the patient as an active participant. In this way the patient feels empowered to be an important part of their own treatment.

CTNA methods can provide a bridge between the provision of diagnostic and educational information and address the dynamics of a patient's family so that they can feel supported and empowered and are active collaborators in the feedback and treatment recommendation process. Clinical experience providing these types of feedback sessions has shown that family members will often confide in the clinician about the need for their own help and support. This provides a segue toward recommendations for family support and care. CTNA methods ensure that information is provided in an open and collaborative way so that participants remain open to the process and the information for their and their loved one's benefit.

Chapter 8
Final Thoughts

As discussed earlier in this book, CTNA challenges practitioners of neuropsychology to broaden the scope of their roles in the assessment process. One of the greatest challenges for the practitioner is the ability to relinquish some level of control of the assessment and feedback process. CTNA empowers patients by making them collaborators and co-interpreters of the assessment results. In addition, they are further empowered to determine the nature and course of outcomes resulting from the assessment. Such a method requires that patients be seen as on an equal footing with the assessor and that their opinions and ideas are of equal importance in determining how to use the neuropsychological information.

Now, someone reading this might be thinking, "So we're supposed to basically give them the information and let them run with it?" The answer to that is, of course, no. That would not be a good practice and would likely be unethical. Any collaborative approach requires finding a delicate balance between using our knowledge, skills, and expertise yet at the same time partnering with patients in a way that views them as experts on themselves. The sets of skills required to create such an atmosphere are not developed by reading a book. Therefore, we have provided some recommendations for learning CTNA skills. These recommendations are for those who have already learned the required skills for conducting and interpreting neuropsychological assessments. Suggested guidelines are put forth from the Houston Conference on Specialty Education and Training in Clinical Neuropsychology (see the American Academy of Clinical Neuropsychology, www.theaacn.org.)

The recommendations presented below are for learning the therapeutic verbal skills of a CTNA session.

1. Read the literature on therapeutic/individualized psychological assessment, specifically the work of Dr. Stephen Finn and Dr. Constance Fischer. References for relevant writings can be found at the end of this book. Their work provides the base from which CTNA methods build.
2. Read the literature on motivational interviewing (MI). It would be highly recommended to read Dr. William Miller and Dr. Steve Rollnick's *Motivational Interviewing: Preparing People to Change*. Additionally, review the MI

T.T. Gorske, S.R. Smith, *Collaborative Therapeutic Neuropsychological Assessment*,   123
DOI: 10.1007/978-0-387-75426-0_8, © Springer Science+Business Media, LLC 2009

website www.motivationalinterview.org. There you will find numerous MI resources. Specifically, you can find the MI bibliography, which includes relevant literature from 1983 to current. On the website, you can also find links to MI learning tools such as their videotape series that reviews all the components of an MI session including special applications in health care.

3. Consider taking a workshop on therapeutic assessment. The annual convention of the Society for Personality Assessment includes numerous seminars and workshops on therapeutic assessment. You can view their website www.personality.org. Also please see Dr. Finn's book *In Our Clients' Shoes: Theory and Techniques of Therapeutic Assessment* for a review of therapeutic assessment methods and suggestions for learning.

4. It would be highly recommended to take at least two workshops on MI principles and methods. In my own (Dr. Gorske's) experience, there are some specific recommendations for learning MI. First would be to take a 2-day basic workshop in order to learn the principles and skills. Next, I would recommend practicing MI skills under the supervision of a MINT trainer. A MINT trainer is a professional who has successfully completed a "Train the Trainer" course in MI. On the MI website, there is a training link that includes names and locations of MINT trainers throughout the world. Next, I would recommend attending a more advanced MI workshop that allows for further structured practice. Finally, I would recommend continual ongoing supervision, including audio or videotape analysis, with a MINT trainer. These are my own (Dr. Gorske's) recommendations based on my own experience as a MINT trainer having trained hundreds of professionals in MI. For further information on suggested MI training methods please see Yahne, Miller, Moyers, and Pirritano (2004).

Finally, it is our sincere hope that readers find this information useful and will consider learning CTNA methods and adopt them in their own clinical practice, teaching, or research. As previously stated, we see CTNA methods as an adjunct to standard neuropsychological testing and assessment methods. We plan to continue using and modifying these methods in our own work and hope others will do the same. In doing so, we would appreciate any opportunities for communication and collaboration as we seek to develop and expand CTNA.

Appendices

In these appendices we have included the following documents for the reader.

1. An abbreviated sample of a CTNA feedback report;
2. Two patient feedback forms; the first is used in clinical practice and the second has been used in research studies;
3. A CTNA adherence scale. This allows clinicians to evaluate their own effectiveness in following CTNA principles and methods.

The reader is welcome to use or modify these documents for their own needs.

Appendix A
Sample CTNA Feedback Report

This is an abbreviated version of the CTNA personalized feedback report. The actual report is approximately 15 pages long, and each page covers a different cognitive test (or series of tests measuring similar functions). However, this form can be adapted and used for any battery of tests an examiner chooses. The reader is welcome to use and adapt this form to meet their own needs.

Neuropsychological Assessment Personal

Feedback Report

Table of Contents

Introduction

Introduction

What is neuropsychology and what is a neuropsychological assessment?

Neuropsychology is the study of how your brain works, which affects your behavior, your thinking, your emotions and feelings, and your overall ability to carry out daily life tasks and routines that allow you to meet life goals.

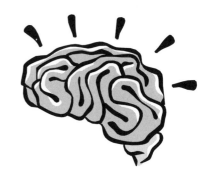

Neuropsychological assessment uses different tests to assess how well you solve problems that require the use of certain skills affected by your brain, your thinking, and your personality.

What skills will the assessment test?

The tests will assess a wide range of skills including your ability to pay attention, concentrate, remember certain information, and solve problems.

What is the personalized feedback report?

The neuropsychological assessment personal feedback report will give you information from the results of the neuropsychological assessments. It will tell you how you scored on each test as compared to other people who have taken the tests.

What kind of information can I expect to learn from the assessment feedback?

The feedback from the neuropsychological assessment will describe the following:

1. Your personal strengths and weaknesses.
2. Reasons related to your thinking and behavior that could explain various problems you are experiencing in your life.
3. Ways your illness or injury may be affecting the skills specified above.
4. The benefits of treatment in improving your thinking and behavior in these skill areas.

Life Implications Section

As part of the feedback report, we would like you to identify some specific questions you hope the test results can answer.

1.

2.

3.

Throughout the feedback report, we will work with you to discover how the skills tested in the neuropsychological assessment have an impact on these life areas you have told us are most important to you.

Your Personal Skill Profile

In the next sections, you will learn which skills are personal strengths and which skills are weaknesses. You will first see a list of your personal strengths followed by a description of how you performed on each test. Your score on each test will be compared to a "standard" score. A standard score is the average score of other people who have taken this test. Your score will fall into one of three categories:

1. **Average**: This means you scored about the same as many people who have taken this test.
2. **Above average**: This means you scored higher as compared to many people who have taken this test.
3. **Below average**: This means you scored lower than many people who have taken this test.

Based on the results of the assessments, here are your strong points, or personal strengths:

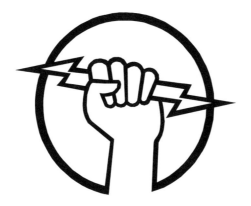

Logical Memory

In a test of your ability to:

- Remember stories/words/phrases that you heard a short time ago and a long time ago.
  - Learn new information that you heard either a short or a long time ago.
    - Focus and pay attention to stories and remember important themes.
      - Recover memories from things that have been told to you.

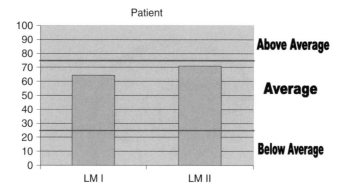

WCST

In a test of your ability to:

- Solve problems,
  - Organize,
    - Use feedback about your performance,
      - Identify and use certain rules and concepts,
        - Be flexible in your thinking.

You performed in the following manner:

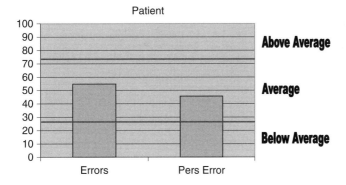

Based on the results of the assessments, here are your challenges or areas of weakness.

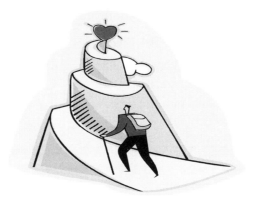

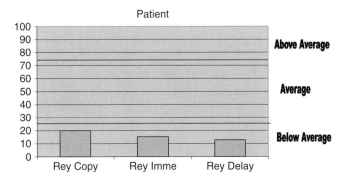

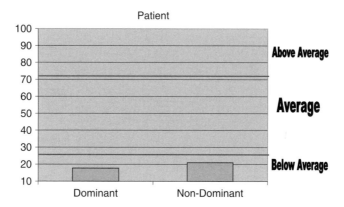

Appendix B
Patient Feedback Form (adapted from Center for Therapeutic Assessment, Austin, Texas)

Strongly disagree	Disagree	Neutral	Agree	Strongly agree
1	2	3	4	5

	Strongly Disagree			Strongly Agree	
1. I felt free to express my thoughts and opinions.	1	2	3	4	5
2. I felt respected as a person.	1	2	3	4	5
3. The session taught me things about myself I didn't know.	1	2	3	4	5
4. I felt free to disagree with the therapist.	1	2	3	4	5
5. The session was a positive experience.	1	2	3	4	5
6. The session captured who I am as a person.	1	2	3	4	5
7. I felt the therapist and I were working together.	1	2	3	4	5
8. I felt I could trust the therapist.	1	2	3	4	5
9. The session made me think about my life.	1	2	3	4	5
10. I had a say in how to use knowledge from the session in my own life.	1	2	3	4	5
11. The therapist was respectful and considerate of my feelings.	1	2	3	4	5
12. Information I learned in the session was applicable to areas of my life I'm concerned about.	1	2	3	4	5
13. The therapist and I worked as a team.	1	2	3	4	5
14. The therapist made me feel important.	1	2	3	4	5
15. The session provided answers to important questions I have about my life.	1	2	3	4	5
16. I helped develop the treatment plan.	1	2	3	4	5
17. I felt judged or criticized during the session.	1	2	3	4	5
18. The treatment plan was suited to my needs and concerns.	1	2	3	4	5
19. The session made me aware of my strengths and weaknesses	1	2	3	4	5

Please make any other comments that you wish us to know on the back of this form.

Appendix C

Patient Feedback Form (**from NAFI pilot study**)

This feedback form is the one used in the NAFI pilot study. It is simpler

and less involved than the previous patient feedback form but can be used and

adapted to fit the needs of the reader.

Instructions: The purpose of neuropsychological assessment is to examine your ability to use skills based on your thinking, emotions, and personality. Such skills include your ability to concentrate, focus, make decisions, problem solve, and remember things. An important part of neuropsychological assessment is the feedback you receive about your performance on the various tests. This feedback should identify your strengths and weaknesses and allow you to work with the examiner to develop understandable and applicable treatment goals. In order to make sure that the feedback is understandable and useful, we would like you to give us feedback on how helpful the testing and feedback was for you.

Please circle the response that most accurately describes your reaction to the question.

1. Overall, what kind of experience was the assessment and feedback session?
   1. Very negative
   2. Negative
   3. Neutral
   4. Positive
   5. Very positive
	5. Did the results of the assessment and feedback apply to daily tasks or problems in your life?
	   1. Not at all
	   2. Very little
	   3. Somewhat
	   4. Very much

2. After the feedback session, did you feel like you understood your problems better?
   1. Not at all
   2. Very little
   3. Somewhat
   4. Very much
	6. Did you understand the feedback that was given to you?
	   1. Not at all
	   2. Very little
	   3. Somewhat
	   4. Very much

3. Did you feel the assessment and feedback accurately identified your strengths?
   1. Not at all
   2. Very little
   3. Somewhat
   4. Very much
	7. Do you believe that the results will motivate you to participate in treatment more fully?
	   1. Not at all
	   2. Very little
	   3. Somewhat
	   4. Very much

4. Do you feel the assessment and feedback accurately identified areas needing improvement?
   1. Not at all
   2. Very little
   3. Somewhat
   4. Very much	

8. Please add any comments stating how the feedback from the assessment was or was not helpful to you in making any changes in your treatment.

_____

_____

_____

_____

_____

Appendix D

CTNA Adherence Scale

Clinician_____   Subject
ID_____

Date_____

Rate quality of the clinician's interventions based on the scale provided below. A score of "1" indicates a low degree of skills, versus a score of "7" indicates a high degree of skill.

Low		High
1.....................3...................................5.....................7		

INTRODUCTION/AGENDA SETTING

_____	Develops the agenda in a collaborative manner by explaining the purpose of the feedback session and eliciting any client questions or concerns.
_____	Introduces the feedback report by asking the client's recollections of the assessment and any reactions they had to completing the tests.
_____	Interacts with the client in an MI-consistent manner using OARS to understand and clarify any client's concerns or perceptions.
_____	Reviews the introduction section and takes time to elicit client reactions. Uses OARS to enhance collaboration.

DEVELOP LIFE IMPLICATIONS QUESTIONS

_____	Elicits client concerns with the life implication questions in specific and concrete terms using OARS.

EXPLAINING PERSONAL SKILL PROFILE (HOW STRENGTHS AND WEAKNESSES ARE DETERMINED

_____	Explains the personal skill profile in simple terms

_____	understandable to the client?

EXPLAINING PERSONAL STRENGTHS AND WEAKNESSES

_____	Reviews personal strengths and weaknesses using Elicit–Provide–Elicit and OARS.
_____	Counselor provides cognitive feedback in an objective and nonjudgmental manner.
_____	When providing information, the counselor explains each cognitive domain in terms understandable to the client?
_____	When providing information, the counselor uses practical, real-life examples to further explain the nature of each cognitive domain?

SUMMARIZING AND MAKING RECOMMENDATIONS

_____	Counselor provides a brief summary of the client's cognitive strengths and weaknesses?
_____	Counselor elicits client's own ideas on how to use this information to make changes in their substance use, psychiatric condition, or other life areas important to the client?
_____	Counselor provides an explanation of the possible relationship between the client's cognitive profile, substance abuse, and psychiatric condition?
_____	Counselor provides information and recommendations for treatment that relates to the feedback results?

References

Ackerman, S. J., Hilsenroth, M. J., Baity, M. R., & Blagys, M. D. (2000) Interaction of therapeutic process and alliance during psychological assessment. *Journal of Personality Assessment, 75*(1), 82–109.

Adams, R. L., Parsons, O. A., Culbertson, J. L., & Nixon, S. J. (Eds.). (1996). *Neuropsychology for clinical practice: Etiology, assessment, and treatment of common neurological disorders.* Washington, DC: American Psychological Association.

Addington, J., & Addington, D. (1997). Substance abuse and cognitive functioning in schizophrenia. *Journal of Psychiatry and Neuroscience, 22*(2), 99–104.

Allen, D. N., Goldstein, G., & Aldarondo, F. (1999). Neurocognitive dysfunction in patients diagnosed with schizophrenia and alcoholism. *Neuropsychology, 13*(1), 62–68.

Allen, J. G., Lewis, L., Blum, S., Voorhees, S., Jernigan, S., & Peebles, M. J. (1986). Informing psychiatric patients and their families about neuropsychological assessment findings. *Bulletin of the Menninger Clinic, 50*(1), 64–74.

American Psychological Association. (2002). Ethical principles of psychologists and code of conduct. *American Psychologist, 57*(12), 1060–1073.

Amrhein, P. C., Miller, W. M., Yahne, C. E., Palmer, M., & Fulcher, L. (2003). Client commitment language during motivational interviewing predicts drug use outcomes. *Journal of Consulting and Clinical Psychology, 71*(5), 862–878.

Armengol, C. G., Kaplan, E., & Moes, E. (Eds.). (2001). *The consumer oriented neuropsychological report.* Lutz, Florida: Psychological Assessment Resources, Inc.

Aronow, E., & Reznikoff, M. (1971). Application of projective tests to psychotherapy: A case study. *Journal of Personality Assessment, 35,* 379–393.

Barrowclough, C., Haddock, G., Tarrier, N., Lewis, S., Moring, J., O'Brien, R., et al. (2001). Randomized controlled trial of motivational interviewing, cognitive behavior therapy, and family intervention for patients with comorbid schizophrenia and substance use disorders. *The American Journal of Psychiatry, 158*(10), 1706–1713.

Bellack, L., Pasquarelli, B. A., & Braverman, S. (1949). The use of the thematic apperception test in psychotherapy. *Journal of Nervous & Mental Disease, 110,* 51–65.

Bem, D. J. (1967). Self-perception: An alternative interpretation of cognitive dissonance phenomena. *Psychological Review, 74,* 183–200.

Bennett-Levy, J., Klein-Boonschate, M. A., Batchelor, J., McCarter, R., & Walton, N. (1994). Encounters with Anna Thompson: The consumer's experience of neuropsychological assessment. *The Clinical Neuropsychologist, 8*(2), 219–238.

Bensing, J. (2000). Bridging the gap. The separate worlds of evidence-based medicine and patient centered medicine. *Patient Education and Counseling, 39*(1), 17–25.

Berg, M. (1984). Expanding the parameters of psychological testing. *Bulletin of the Menninger Clinic, 48*(1), 10–24.

Berg, M. (1985). The feedback process in diagnostic psychological testing. *Bulletin of the Menninger Clinic, 49*(1), 52–69.

Bien, T. H., Miller, W. R., & Boroughs, J. M. (1993). Motivational Interviewing with alcohol outpatients. *Behavioural and Cognitive Psychotherapy*, 21, 347–356.

Blume, A. W., Davis, J. M., & Schmaling, K. B. (1999). Neurocognitive dysfunction in dually-diagnosed patients: A potential roadblock to motivating behavior change. *Journal of Psychoactive Drugs*, 31(2), 111–115.

Boake, C. (1989). A history of cognitive rehabilitation of head-injured patients, 1915 to 1980. *Journal of Head Trauma Rehabilitation*, 4(3), 1–8.

Book, H. (1998). *Socialization interview*. In H. Book (Ed.), *How to practice brief psychodynamic psychotherapy: The core conflictual relationship theme method* (pp. 101–107), 181 pp. Washington, DC, US: American Psychological Association.

Brodsky, S. (1972). Shared results and open files with the client. *Professional Psychology*, 3, 362–364.

Brown, F. M. & Wiggins, J. G. (2005). A survey of clinicians' practices with older adults. In M. Storandt & G. VandenBos (Eds.), *Neuropsychological assessment of dementia and depression in older adults: A clinician's guide* (pp. 177–181). Washington, DC: American Psychological Association.

Carpenter, K. M., & Hittner, J. B. (1997). Cognitive impairment among the dually diagnosed: Substance use history and depressive symptom correlates. *Addiction*, 92(6), 747–759.

Carroll, K. M., Libby, B., Sheehan, J., & Hyland, N. (2001). Motivational interviewing to enhance treatment initiation in substance abusers: An effectiveness study. *The American Journal on Addictions*, 10, 335–339.

Casey, J. E., Strang, J. D., Roach, D. A., & Innerd, W. L. (1997). The neuropsychology case conference: A model for providing assessment feedback. *The Clinical Neuropsychologist*, 11, 302.

Christensen, A. L. (1975). *Luria's neuropsychological investigation*. New York: Spectrum Publications, Inc.

Christensen, A. L., & Caetano, C. (1996). Aleksandr Romanovich Luria (1902–1977): Contributions to neuropsychological rehabilitation. *Neuropsychological Rehabilitation*, 6(4), 279–303.

Christensen, A. L., & Caetano, C. (1999a). Luria's neuropsychological investigation in the Nordic countries. *Neuropsychology Review*, 9(2), 71–78.

Christensen, A. L., & Caetano, C. (1999b). Neuropsychological rehabilitation in the interdisciplinary team: The post acute stage. In D. T. Stuss, G. Winocur, & I. H. Robertson (Eds.), *Cognitive neurorehabilitation* (pp. 188–200). Cambridge: Cambridge University Press.

Cicerone, K. D., Dahlberg, C., Malec, J. F., Langenbahn, D. M., Felicetti, T., Kneipp, S., Ellmo, W., Kalmar, K., Giacino, J. T., Harley, J. P., Laatsch, L., Morse, P. A., & Catanese, J. (2005). Evidence-based cognitive rehabilitation: Updated review of the literature from 1998 through 2002. *Archives of Physical Medicine and Rehabilitation*, 86, 1681–1692.

Cronbach, L. J. (1949). *Essentials of psychological testing*. New York: Harper & Brothers.

Crosson, B., Barco, P. P., Velozo, C. A., Bolesta, M. M., Cooper, P. V., Werts, D., & Brobeck, T. C. (1989). Awareness and compensation in postacute head injury rehabilitation. *Journal of Head Trauma Rehabilitation*, 4(3), 46–54.

Crosson, B. (2000). Application of neuropsychological assessment results. In R. D. Vanderploeg (Ed.), *Clinician's guide to neuropsychological assessment* (2nd ed., pp. 195–244). Mahwah: Lawrence Erlbaum Associates.

Daley, D. C., Salloum, I. M., Zuckoff, A., Kirisci, L., & Thase, M. E. (1998). Increasing treatment adherence among outpatients with depression and cocaine dependence: Results of a pilot study. *American Journal of Psychiatry*, 155(11), 1611–1613.

Dana, R. H., & Leech, S. (1974). Existential assessment. *Journal of Personality Assessment*, 38, 428–435.

DiClemente, C., Marinilli, A., Singh, M., & Bellino, L. (2001). The role of feedback in the process of health behavior change. *American Journal of Health Behavior*, 25(3), 217–227.

Donofrio, N., Piatt, A., Whelihan, W., & DiCarlo, M. (1999). Neuropsychological test feedback: Consumer evaluation and perceptions. *Archives of Clinical Neuropsychology*, 14(8), 721.

Festinger, L. (1957). *A theory of cognitive dissonance*. Stanford, CA: Stanford University Press.

Finn, S. E., & Tonsager, M. E. (1992). Therapeutic effects of providing MMPI-2 test feedback to college students awaiting therapy. *Psychological Assessment*, 4(3), 278–287.

Finn, S. E. (1996a). Assessment and feedback integrating MMPI-2 and rorschach findings. *Journal of Personality Assessment*, 67(3), 543–557.

Finn, S. E. (1996b). *Using the MMPI-2 as a therapeutic intervention*. Minneapolis: University of Minnesota Press.

Finn, S. E. & Martin, H. (1997). Therapeutic assessment with the MMPI-2 in managed health care. In J. N. Butcher (Ed.), *Objective personality assessment in managed care: A practitioner's guide* (pp.131–152). New York: Oxford University Press.

Finn, S. E., & Tonsager, M. E. (1997). Information gathering and therapeutic models of assessment: complementary paradigms. *Psychological Assessment*, 9(4), 374–385.

Finn, S. E., & Tonsager, M. E. (2002). How therapeutic assessment became humanistic. *The Humanistic Psychologist*, 30, 10–22.

Finn, S. E. (2003). Therapeutic assessment of a Man with "ADD". *Journal of Personality Assessment*, 80(2), 115–129.

Finn, S. E., & Kamphuis, J. H. (2006). Therapeutic assessment with the MMPI-2. In J. N. Butcher (Ed.), *MMPI-2: A practitioner's guide*. Washington, DC: APA Books.

Finn, S.E. (2007). *In our client's shoes: Theory and techniques of therapeutic assessment*. Mahwah, NJ: Lawrence Erlbaum Associates.

Fischer, C. T. (1970). The testee as co-evaluator. *Journal of Counseling Psychology*, 17(1), 70–76.

Fischer, C. T. (1972). Paradigm changes which allow sharing of results. *Professional Psychology*, 3, 364–369.

Fischer, C. T. (1979). Individualized assessment and phenomenolgical psychology. *Journal of Personality Assessment*, 43(2), 115–122.

Fischer, C. T. (1994). *Individualizing psychological assessment* (2nd ed.). Hillsdale, NJ: Lawrence Erlbaum Associates.

Fischer, C. T. (2000). Collaborative, Individualized Assessment. *Journal of Personality Assessment*, 74(1), 2–14.

Fischer, C. T. (2003). Infusing humanistic perspectives into psychology. *Journal of Humanistic Psychology*, 43(3), 93–105.

Fischer, C. T., & Finn, S. E. (2008). Developing life meaning from psychological test data: Collaborative and therapeutic approaches. In R. P. Archer & S.R. Smith (Eds.), *Personality assessment* (pp. 379–404). New York: Routledge.

Flach, S. D., McCoy, K. D., Vaughn, T. E., Ward, M. M., Bootsmiller, B. J., & Doebbeling, B. N. (2004). Does patient-centered care improve provision of preventive services? *Journal of General Internal Medicine*, 19(10), 1019–1026.

Fleming, J., & Strong, J. (1995). Self awareness of deficits following acquired brain injury: Considerations for rehabilitation. *British Journal of Occupational Therapy*, 98, 55–60.

Gass, C. S., & Brown, M. C. (1992). Neuropsychological test feedback to patients with brain dysfunction. *Psychological Assessment*, 4(3), 272–277.

Gordon, W. A., Zafonte, R., Cicerone, K., Cantor, J., Brown, M., Lombard, L., et al. (2006). Traumatic brain injury rehabilitation: State of the science. *American Journal of Physical Medicine and Rehabilitation*, 85, 343–382.

Gorske, T. (2008). Therapeutic neuropsychological assessment: A humanistic model and case example. *Journal of Humanistic Psychology*, 48(3), 320–339.

Green, J. (2000). *Neuropsychological evaluation of the older adult: A clinicians' handbook*. San Diego: Academic Press.

Groth-Marnat, G. (1999a). Current status and future directions of psychological assessment: Introduction. *Journal of Clinical Psychology*, 55(7), 781–785.

Groth-Marnat, G. (1999b). Financial efficacy of clinical assessment: rational guidelines and issues for future research. *Journal of Clinical Psychology*, 55(7), 813–824.

Groth-Marnat, G. (2000). Visions of clinical assessment: Then, now, and a brief history of the future. *Journal of Clinical Psychology*, 56(3), 349–365.

Groth-Marnat, G. (2003). *Handbook of psychological assessment* (4th ed.). Hoboken: Wiley.

Handler, L., & Hilsenroth, M. (Eds.). (1998). *Teaching and learning personality assessment*. Mahwah, NJ: Lawrence Erlbaum Associates.

Handler, L., & Meyer, G.J. (1998). The importance of teaching and learning personality assessment. In L. Handler & M.J. Hilsenroth (Eds.), *Teaching and learning personality assessment*. Mahwah, NJ: Lawrence Erlbaum Associates, Inc.

Harrower, M. (1956). Projective counseling: A psychotherapeutic technique. *American Journal of Psychotherapy*, 10, 74–86.

Heitler, J. (1973). Preparation of lower-class patients for expressive group psychotherapy. *Journal of Consulting and Clinical Psychology*, 41(2), 251–260.

Hester, R. K., Squires, D. D., & Delaney, H. D. (2005). The drinkers checkup: 12 month outcomes of a controlled clinical trial of a stand-alone software program for problem drinkers. *Journal of Substance Abuse Treatment*, 28, 159–169.

Hettema, J., Steele, J., & Miller, W. M. (2005). Motivational Interviewing. *Annual Review of Psychology*, 1, 91–111.

Hilsenroth, M., Peters, E., & Ackerman, S. (2004). The development of therapeutic alliance during psychological assessment: Patient and therapist perspectives across treatment. *Journal of Personality Assessment*, 83(3), 332–344.

Horvath, A., & Symonds, D. (1991). Relation between working alliance and outcome in psychotherapy: A meta-analysis. *Journal of Counseling Psychology*, 38(2), 139–149.

Fletcher-Janzen, E., Strickland, T., & Reynolds, C. (2000). *Handbook of cross-cultural neuropsychology*. New York: Kluwer Academic/Plenum Publishers.

Katz, N., Fleming, J., Keren, N., Lightbody, S., & Hartman-Maeir, A. (2002). Unawareness and/or denial of disability: Implications for occupational therapy intervention. *Canadian Journal for Occupational Therapy*, 69, 281–292.

Katz, D., Ashley, M., O'Shanick, G., & Connors, S. (2006). *Cognitive rehabilitation: The evidence, funding, and case for advocacy in brain injury*. McLean, VA: Brain Injury Association of America.

Klonoff, P., Watt, L., Dawson, L., Henderson, S., Gehrels, J., & Wethe, J. (2006). Psychosocial outcomes 1–7 years after comprehensive milieu-oriented neurorehabilitation: The role of pre-injury status. *Brain Injury*, 20(6), 601–612.

Knight, B. (2005). Providing clinical interpretations to older clients and their families. In Storandt, M., & VandenBos, G. (Eds.), *Neuropsychological assessment of dementia and depression in older adults: A clinician's guide*. Washington, DC: American Psychological Association.

Lewak, R.W., & Hogan, R.S. (2003). Integrating and applying assessment information: Decision making, patient feedback, and consultation. In L. E. Beutler & G. Groth-Marnat (Eds.), *Integrative assessment of adult personality* (pp. 356–397). New York: Guilford.

Lezak, M. D., Howieson, D. B., & Loring, D. W. (2004). *Neuropsychological assessment* (4th ed.). New York: Oxford University Press.

Luborsky, L. (1953). Self-interpretation of the TAT as a clinical technique. *Journal of Projective Techniques*, 17, 217–223.

Luborsky, L. (1984). *Principles of psychoanalytic psychotherapy: A manual for Supportive – Expressive (SE) treatment*. New York: Basic Books.

Luria, A. R. (1966). *Higher cortical functions in man*. New York: Basic Books.

Luria, A. R. (1972). *The man with the shattered world: The history of a brain wound*. Cambridge, MA: Harvard University Press.

Malla, A. K., Lazosky, A., McLean, T., Rickwood, A., Cheng, S., & Norman, R. M. G. (1997). Neuropsychological assessment as an aid to psychosocial rehabilitation in severe mental disorders. *Psychiatric Rehabilitation Journal*, 21(2), 169–173.

Martin, D.J., Garske, J.P., & Davis, M.K. (2000) Relation of the therapeutic alliance with outcome and other variables: A meta-analytic review. *Journal of Consulting and Clinical Psychology*, 68, 438–450.

Martino, S., Carroll, K. M., O'Malley, S., & Rounsaville, B. J. (2000). Motivational interviewing with psychiatrically ill substance abusing patients. *The American Journal on Addictions*, 9, 88–91.

Mead, N., & Bower, P. (2000). Patient-centredness: A conceptual framework and review of the empirical literature. *Social Science and Medicine*, 51, 1087–1110.

Meek, P. S., Clark, H. W., & Solana, V. (1989). Neurocognitive impairment: The unrecognized component of dual diagnosis in substance abuse treatment. *Journal of Psychoactive Drugs*, 21(2), 153–160.

Meyer, G. J., Finn, S. E., Eyde, L. D., Kay, G. G., Moreland, K. L, Dies, R. R., Eisman, E. J., Kubiszyn, T. W., & Reed, G. M. (2001). Psychological testing and psychological assessment: A review of evidence and issues. *American Psychologist*, 56(2), 128–165.

Michel, D. M. (2002). Psychological assessment as a therapeutic intervention in patients hospitalized with eating disorders. *Professional Psychology: Research and Practice*, 33(5), 470–477.

Miller, W. M., Sovereign, R. G., & Krege, B. (1988). Motivational interviewing with problem drinkers: II. The drinkers checkup as a preventative intervention. *Psychotherapy*, 16, 251–268.

Miller, W. R., Zweben, A., DiClemente, C. C., & Rychtarik, R. G. (1992). *Motivational enhancement therapy manual: A clinical research guide for therapists treating individuals with alcohol abuse and dependence*. Rockville, MD: National Institute on Alcohol Abuse and Alcoholism.

Miller, W. R., Benefield, R. G., & Tonigan, J. S. (1993). Enhancing motivation for change in problem drinking: A controlled comparison of two therapist styles. *Journal of Consulting and Clinical Psychology*, 61(3), 455–461.

Miller, W. R., & Rollnick, S. (1991, 2002). *Motivational interviewing: Preparing people to change*. New York: Guilford Press.

Mosak, H. H., & Gushurst, R. S. (1972). Some therapeutic uses of psychological testing. *American Journal of Psychotherapy*, 26, 539–546.

Moyers, T. B., & Rollnick, S. (2002). A motivational interviewing perspective on resistance in psychotherapy. *Journal of Clinical Psychology*, 58, 185–193.

National Institute of Health consensus development panel on rehabilitation of persons with traumatic brain injury. (1999). Rehabilitation of persons with traumatic brain injury. *Journal of the American Medical Association*, 282(10), 974–983.

Newman, M. L., & Greenway, P. (1997). Therapeutic effects of providing MMPI-2 test feedback to clients at a university counseling service: A collaborative approach. *Psychological Assessment*, 9(2), 122–131.

Nixon, S. J., Hallford, G., & Tivis, R. D. (1996). Neurocognitive functioning in alcoholic, schizophrenic and dually diagnosed patients. *Psychiatry Research*, 64, 35–45.

Pegg, P., Auerbach, S., Seel, R., Buenaver, L., Kiesler, D., & Plybon, L. (2005). The impact of patient-centered information on patients' treatment satisfaction and outcomes in traumatic brain injury rehabilitation. *Rehabilitation Psychology*, 50(4), 366–374.

Pope, K. S. (1992). Responsibilities in providing psychological test feedback to clients. *Psychological Assessment*, 4(3), 268–271.

Prigatano, G. (1999). *Principles of neuropsychological rehabilitation*. New York: Oxford University Press, Inc.

Prochaska, J. O., DiClemente, C. C., & Norcross, J. C. (1992). In search of how people change: Applications to addictive behaviors. *American Psychologist*, 47, 1102–1114.

Reis, B., & Brown, L. (1999). Reducing psychotherapy dropouts: Maximizing perspective convergence in the psychotherapy dyad. *Psychotherapy: Theory/Research/Practice/Training*, 36, 123–136.

Resnicow, K., DiLorio, C., Soet, J. E., Borelli, B., Hecht, J., & Ernst, D. (2002). Motivational interviewing in health promotion: It sounds like something is changing. *Health Psychology*, 21(5), 444–451.

Rogers, C. R. (1942). *Counseling and psychotherapy*. Boston: Houghton Mifflin.

Rogers, C. R. (1951). *Client-centered therapy*. Boston: Houghton Mifflin.

Ruff, R. (2003). A friendly critique of neuropsychology: Facing the challenges of our future. *Archives of Clinical Neuropsychology*, 18(8), 847–864.

Schönberger, M., Humle, F., Zeeman, P., & Teasdale, T. (2006). Patient compliance in brain injury rehabilitation in relation to awareness and cognitive and physical improvement. *Neuropsychological Rehabilitation*, 16(5), 561–578.

Schönberger, M., Humle, F., Zeeman, P., & Teasdale, T. (2006). Working alliance and patient compliance in brain injury rehabilitation and their relation to psychosocial outcome. *Neuropsychological Rehabilitation*, 16(3), 298–314.

Serper, M. R., Bergman, A., & Copersino, M. L. (2000). Learning and memory impairment in cocaine dependent and comorbid schizophrenic patients. *Psychiatry Research*, 93, 21–32.

Smith, S., Wiggins, C., & Gorske, T. (2007). A survey of psychological assessment feedback practices. *Assessment*, 14(3), 310–319.

Storandt, M., & VandenBos, G. (2005). *Neuropsychological assessment of dementia and depression in older adults: A clinician's guide*. Washington, DC: American Psychological Association.

Stotts, A., Schmitz, J. M., Rhoades, H. M., & Grabowski, J. (2001). Motivational interviewing with cocaine-dependent patients: A pilot study. *Journal of Consulting and Clinical Psychology*, 69(5), 858–862.

Strang, J. D. (1987). Educational and related treatment considerations with the epileptic child: A developmental neuropsychological approach. In A. P. Aldenkamp, W. C. J. Alpert, H. Meinardi, & G. Stores (Eds.), *Education and epilepsy: Proceedings of an international workshop on education in epilepsy*, (pp. 118–1345). Amsterdam: Swets & Zeitlinger.

Swanson, A. J., Pantalon, M. V., & Cohen, K. R. (1999). Motivational interviewing and treatment adherence among psychiatric and dually diagnosed patients. *Journal of Nervous & Mental Disease*, 187(10), 630–636.

Tharinger, D. J., Finn, S. E., Wilkinson, A. D., & Schaber, P. M. (2007). Therapeutic Assessment with a child as a family intervention: Clinical protocol and research case study. *Psychology in the Schools,* 44(3), 293–309.

Tracy, J. I., Josiassen, R. C., & Bellack, A. S. (1995). Neuropsychology of dual diagnosis: Understanding the combined effects of schizophrenia and substance use disorders. *Clinical Psychology Review*, 15(2), 67–97.

Van den Broek, M.D. (2005). Why does neurorehabilitation fail? *Journal of Head Trauma Rehabilitation*, 20(5), 464–473.

Walters, S. T., & Neighbors, C. (2005). Feedback interventions for college alcohol misuse: What, why and for whom? *Addictive Behaviors*, 30, 1168–1182.

Wampold, B. (2001). *The great psychotherapy debate: Models, methods, and findings*. Mahwah, NJ: Lawrence Erlbaum Associates Inc.

Wolff, W. (1956). *Contemporary psychotherapists examine themselves*. Springfield, IL: Charles C. Thomas.

Yahne, C. E., Miller, W. R., Moyers, T. B., & Pirritano, M. A randomized trial of methods to help clinician's learn Motivational Interviewing. *Journal of Consulting and Clinical Psychology*, 72(6), 1050–1062.

Zandbelt, L., Smets, E., Oort, F., Haes, H. (2005). Coding patient-centred behaviour in the medical encounter. *Social Science and Medicine*, 61, 661–671.

Zandbelt, L., Smets, E., Oort, F., Godfried, M., & de Haes, H. (2007). Medical specialists' patient centered communication and patient-reported outcomes. *Medical Care*, 45(4), 330–339.

Index

Printed in the United States of America